LECTURES, TUTORIALS AND THE LIKE

LECTURES, TUTORIALS AND THE LIKE

A Primer in the Techniques of
Higher Scientific Education

DR. A. J. WALTON

MTP

Medical and Technical Publishing Co Ltd
Oxford and Lancaster
1972

Published by

MTP

Medical and Technical Publishing Co Ltd
Seacourt Tower, Oxford and
St. Leonard's House, Lancaster

Copyright © 1972 by Dr. A. J. Walton
Softcover reprint of the hardcover 1st 1972

ISBN-13: 978-94-011-6125-1   e-ISBN-13: 978-94-011-6123-7
DOI: 10.1007/978-94-011-6123-7

First Published 1972

Preface

The main qualification which I boast for writing this book is that I have sat through some ten years of university lectures. As a result of this experience I feel like relieving my soul. Not that I anticipate standards will be raised by my doing so, but rather that someone important and helpful will be driven to break silence. Silence it is, for, with few exceptions, nothing appears to have been done to help the new graduate lecturer to face his first audience. Search the libraries and you will find books on how to deal with rowdy secondary school children, with adults who wish to make coffee tables, with the mentally handicapped. But with 'students'? Never. Well, hardly ever. To be honest, I did find a short booklet entitled *The Art of Lecturing* by Dr G. Kitson Clark and Commander E. Bidder Clark, published by Heffers. This, I like to think, helped me. But it was primarily directed at the arts man and much of it did not ring true amidst the clatter of test tubes. So I offer these thoughts realising that they, in turn, are unlikely to disturb any whose business is with the arts!

Although the compulsion to write this book arose from my experiences within the confines of university cloisters I am sure that similar problems arise wherever science is taught; be it in Technical College, Polytechnic, College of Education, Industrial Training Centre or in schools. Whilst the locale may differ, our common concern is to keep our heads above water. Too many of us are thrown in at the deep end and left to flounder. Of course I realise that there are numerous in-depth studies of student learning processes but, let me confess it, I found these singularly unhelpful while nervously waiting to take the plunge. Consequently, my own advice is, frankly, downright earthy!

Notwithstanding educational theorists (who are all-too-frequently arts men), I take it as axiomatic that the existing pattern of lectures, tutorials, practicals, etc., common throughout higher scientific education, will persist for some time to come.

A special word of thanks is due to Pearline Daniels, not only for translating my scrawl into typescript, but for the many helpful noises made at appropriate times. Peter Horrobin also made many helpful comments. My thanks go to him and, indeed, to all those colleagues who had their say.

Alan J. Walton   April 1970

Contents

	PREFACE	v
1	What they expect	1
2	Course planning	5
3	Lecture writing	13
4	The world première	21
5	On stage	31
6	The blackboard	41
7	Screened	49
8	Demonstrations	61
9	Tutorials	73
10	Seminars, colloquia, symposia, and such-like	83
11	Conferences	90
12	Facing the music	98
	Bibliography	104

*to all those who provoked
me into taking up my pen*

CHAPTER

1

What they expect

Come this September it will be nine years since we forsook the world. Three years squandered on a B.Sc., three years devoted to a Ph.D., and three years honoured with a Fellowship which is about to be terminated. Not to put too fine an edge on it, we have been on the lookout for a job. We have, of course, looked the world over and found it lacking. It was never designed with us in view. Anyway it has got its standards hopelessly mixed up; it just doesn't appreciate proper qualifications. We are particularly highly qualified. Particularly highly qualified, if you must know, to stay put. Which explains why Lectureships exist and why we have just been awarded one.

There is a subtle distinction between a Fellowship and a Lectureship. But in July, with term some three months away, the distinction seems unduly subtle. Life is all roses and beer. August arrives, we examine the etymological origins of lectureship, and recall that a new assistant lecturer took us in our first term at university. We have lived to regret the uncharitable thoughts we once harboured against him. We were somewhat hasty in our judgment, were we not? A trifle unsympathetic too when we remember that he was fresh from being a student himself. No one gave him any training.

By mid-September the time has come for action, particularly now that time-tables are blossoming forth bearing our names. So, with the last rose of summer we go to our professors, and say 'Give us some training'. And what do they reply? 'No training given.' The unmistakable inference is that you and I shouldn't need it. Well then, if that is their reaction we will argue that lectures may not be a good thing after all. We will convince them that programmed texts are more eloquent than we could ever be. That good films are more worth watching than us. That we could use tapes from other universities. That . . . No, better not at this stage. They might infer we are trying to run away from things, and it would never do to give that impression. Such thoughts can wait until after we have finished our first lecture course. Then they will agree with us.

Let us take stock. Just what have we been up to these past six years? Why, we have been doing research; pushing back the frontiers; opening up new horizons. Call it what you will, we have been making the world a better place for our children. And for their children. We have also made many sacrifices. Our novel reading, our theatre-going, even our personal virtues, have all gone on the altar. Everyone who has not our exact interests is a bore. We need not lay the blame wholly at our own doors. Pressing research supervisors, the liquid helium that will last for twenty-three hours; the bacteria which (like our kids) insist on being fed at 2.00 a.m.; the stars that refuse to appear by day, have all played their part. True we can now give any of our ex-friends no end of details about the $P_{\frac{3}{2}}$ energy levels of iridium washed down with 1-2-dimethylbenzene. All good solid stuff, mind you. The sort of stuff which guarantees that we are at long last qualified to teach a class of several hundred first-year undergraduates how to solve a quadratic; pull a bunsen-burner to bits; hatch a tadpole, or whatever it is they expect of us. The sort of stuff which guarantees that we know how to expound to perfection on the tadpole, the bunsen-burner, or the quadratic.

And what of those who will sit at our feet? What brings them here? Have they heard of us, and of our work on the $P_{\frac{3}{2}}$ energy levels in iridium? No, they are coming here for strictly non-academic reasons. They have been sold the university by that colour-supplement feature; by that attractively printed prospectus with its views of the snack-bar and the library taken early one Monday morning; and by saucy sixth-form gossip. It's true that some may have been stimulated by watching our professor supplement his salary every Monday evening at 11.15 p.m. on B.B.C.1 for the past six months. Some may even have been favourably influenced on learning that the top professor, who never appears, has earned himself a dukedom for his research students' services. But will they be having the Duke? Yes, for their first lecture. Then it will be the likes of us. Us who haven't even scraped an F.R.S., let alone a knighthood. However, it is a fact that our work on the $P_{\frac{3}{2}}$ levels in iridium has been published in *The Proceedings of the Littlepool Physical Society (Section A)* 78, 137 and we have had requests for seven, repeat seven, reprints out of the five hundred we ordered. If anyone sounds sceptical, we will show him the request cards carefully filed away. And once the paper has been abstracted in *Physics Abstracts,* which we calculate should happen next month, we shall have a further flood of requests. Consoling ourselves that even the Duke must have begun like this, we await our turn.

The Duke's lecture didn't really count. It was largely reminiscent. He has been reminiscing for the past twenty-five years. He can. He told them not to bother taking any notes as he merely wanted to whet their appetites for what was to follow. (Or so they thought.) The old charlatan somehow caught their imaginations. He made everything sound so easy, so trivially easy. Then all those stories about the subject being mathematical were unfounded. Oh yes, they excused the fool's hesitant delivery, his fumbling for words. His meanderings only further increased their fascination. After all, it is not every day that you meet the self-same person who suggested to Einstein that E might just equal mc^2. Or the person who said 'Try this, sir' to Lister when all else had failed. And they believed every word of it. With ten minutes to go, the Duke looked at his watch and sailed out on a burst of applause, leaving the field wide open for us. Ten to one he doesn't even know our names.

What will they make of our groping around for words? Will our meanderings fascinate them? Of course we could tell how we once worked in the same laboratory as Ken Smith and of the day that Maynard-Smith bought us a drink. And that's the truth. But their names will mean nothing. Besides, we don't even look the part. If we did we might try bluffing them. But we don't.

We awake hoping it won't be so.

2

Course planning

It's inevitable. Some time before the fateful October, a letter will arrive informing you that you, yes you, Alan John Walton, have been selected to give the introductory course on 'The relativistic wave-mechanics of second-order pion-pion scattering'. Three possible courses of action are now open to you.

1. Write and tender your resignation

This may be ruled out as three months' salary is normally required in lieu of notice.

2. Have a skim through your own undergraduate notes

You never know, you may have been lucky enough to have had a course of lectures on the subject from your old professor. But tread carefully. The danger is that in adopting his notes you may, quite unwittingly, deal with only the first-order breed of things. Or his treatment may have been non-relativistic. While such deficiencies are unlikely to cause you sleepless nights, even if you spot them, there will always be one student in the class who does understand these matters. He will become very hot under his non-existent collar and will make a great song and dance about lecturers who forget their briefs. So this source of wisdom is best left untapped. Besides there is a distinct possibility that your professor got his notes from his professor and that, if discreet enough enquiries were to be made, the whole thing could be traced back to Lucretius (who is considered rather square today).

3. Get hold of a copy of a simple dictionary of science and try to find out what it's all about

Don't try and do too much to begin with. Just get the general discipline cleared up. Is it to do with astronomy or bacteriology? No? Well then, how about physics? Correct, but you must not rest on your laurels; more will be expected of you than this. If you look up a specialist dictionary you will, however, discover that you have been asked to lecture on nuclear physics. You are almost home and dry. All you require are the catalogues of every publisher. Someone, somewhere, must have written a work entitled *The Relativistic Wave-Mechanics of Second-Order Pion-Pion Scattering*. It is your job to discover who. I need scarcely say that you must now copy the book out word for word, then burn it, and suppress the title. You will recommend every other book in the land on subjects from animal husbandry to zoanthropy before this one. You must disclose to no one, no, not even your nearest and dearest, that the roots of your learning lie in *The Relativistic Wave-Mechanics of Second-Order Pion-Pion Scattering* by one J. R. Slyn-Boyle. Though make a better job of it than did the lecturers of your youth. Remember that course you attended where the source was inadequately suppressed? Remember how, browsing one day in a bookshop, you landed on the fountain where it all came from? Remember how you eagerly turned the pages to glean what topic he would tackle next? How you laughed when he couldn't copy it out correctly, and how you roared when the only problems he attempted were those worked out in the text. And the fool went on living in his little paradise. No, the obliteration must be complete. You must scour every bookshop and every library for copies, remove these and scatter them to the four winds. Sign agreements with the publishers to purchase every copy they intend printing from now to eternity. Search out and obliterate; that must be your motto. And if you are still determined to press on relentlessly, then ponder this. The time; three centuries ago. A solitary scholar winds his lonely way to Cambridge where, neath flickering candle with quill in hand, he doth make fair copy on vellum of some priceless manuscript. The which he doth now digest. And it entered your head to cog something out of the nearest textbook ten minutes before the lecture is due to begin? Then rushing in, you will scrawl it on to the blackboard mutilating it as you go while they, scribbling it down in their Woolworth's jotters, mutilate it still further. And would they ever look at it again? Reflect long and deep on this and ask yourself just what higher education has been up to these past three centuries. And if you remain unrepentant, do at least be honest. Say: 'To-day's lecture is taken from the second chapter of the first book of Slyn-Boyle the physicist, entitled *The Relativistic Wave-Mechanics of Second-Order Pion-Pion Scattering*, be-gining to read at the first equation.' Admit that it's the only text you can afford, that it's the only one you can vaguely comprehend, and that you could not possibly improve on it. But don't query why lectures are held.

Possessing intellectual integrity like ours has its draw-backs: we have just landed ourselves with the task of having to compose a course of lectures. We are too damn honest, that's our failing. But no going back; we will ask the old hands what we should do.

You and I must first do some general reading. Appar-ently there is little point in preparing a course on ecology if we think the Beagle is still in port: our ignorance will show through. Likewise a course of lectures on pions will sound singularly unconvincing if you are still under the impression that phlogiston explains all, because it doesn't. This general reading will take you back to where you were six years ago. It must be followed with up-to-date, more specialised material. Of course, it's tough going, but you are only supposed to be fishing around for ideas at this stage, so skip the fine details. This little exercise is planned, in the words of a professor of education, to encourage you to 'know your subject thoroughly', and is generally number one on any educationalist's list of priorities. Pure therapy designed to blow away the cobwebs and make you come over all of a sparkle. Unless you are better genned up than Einstein was, the class will seeth with the rumour that you are not his equal, and you and your pions will be quickly discounted. There's your motivation!

Too much idealism can prove very dangerous at this juncture. You may awaken one morning wondering why the hell anyone should wish to know about *E. coli* growth media, or why pions have second-order interactions. With millions starving in the world today, what right have I to devote myself to such trifles? A good question. Try writing to the director of some charity or to the professor who dreamt up this course. Better still, read a book on educational objectives. If that doesn't quieten you down, then try a course of self-hypnosis. 'All my life I have cared passionately for *E. coli*. From the cradle upwards, my only love has been *E. coli*. To my dying day I will cherish *E. coli* close to my bosom. Even after.' Three times a day before meals. And if that doesn't do the trick, nothing will. A subject which bores you is unlikely to excite your audience.

With everything proceeding to plan, a collection of possible topics should have formed in your head. You can hardly help it. Now write these ideas down as a series of headings and ask yourself these questions.

1. Whose shoes am I wearing?

Perhaps the easiest trap to walk into is to plan the course of lectures *you* would like to hear; not even the course you would have appreciated as an undergraduate, and that is no commendation, but the course you, with all your superior knowledge, would enjoy right now. The ground is particularly treacherous if you have, for example, been told to lecture a mob of engineers on your passion – fungi. You will find it hard to credit, but engineers don't care a damn about

fungi. If they are stimulated by anything outside of the nurses' home, it is by something like bridge design. But the powers-that-be have decided (as powers-that-be are disposed to decide) that engineers must study mycology, because engineers have always studied mycology, and because employers take it for granted that our graduates can speak the language. So be it. Your job is to awaken the love of fungi which lies dormant in everyone, even in engineers. According to the theorists you have simply to tell them some tall story about slimes on Sydney Harbour Bridge and, before the week is out, they will all be growing mushrooms in their digs. Frankly, these *service courses* are very difficult to prepare. They stand little hope of success, unless you are at least sympathetic towards the student's professed major interest. Ideally you should attend the lectures on their major subject, but studying the syllabus or inspecting their time-table may be a salutary enough experience to put some of your suggested topics in proper perspective. One thing is very certain; you need not expect to motivate students by announcing: 'You won't see the relevance of this now, but you will in five years' time', although stating this much may be preferable to offering no excuses. So we now have a selection of topics which should fire them in their shoes, if anything will.

2. Have I a realistic number of headings?

Most lecturers, especially in planning their first course, wildly over-estimate the amount of material they can get through. It's a pretty safe bet that you have over-estimated this by a factor of two. In plain English, you have material for twice as many lectures as you have been allocated! Omit to halve the number now and by Christmas you will be in such a flap that you will be leaving out all the important topics, which are the ones that take the time. Instead you will pass your remaining days chatting generally about 'biology', nonchalantly suggesting to the class that they

'might care to look up one or two things' for themselves.
They won't care to.

3. How much should I assume?

Nothing, is the short answer. Almost all our profession go
to the other extreme and assume their listeners have heard
it all many times before. They mistake the chuckling of a
totally bewildered audience with the cooing of an understanding class. The chuckles only encourage the belief that
their wisdom is falling on fertile ground, so they plough
ever deeper and deeper. A great *esprit de corps*, an excellent
quality in itself, develops in the class who find the lecturer's
earnestness ever more to their liking. It's a cumulative
process only brought down to earth in the seventh week of
the course on 'Fourier Transforms' when the spokesman,
pointing at an integral sign, asks: 'Please sir, what does the
squiggle represents?' Such lecturers then fill with remorse
and lay on extra classes to teach them how to solve quadratic
equations. Fourier's name is never breathed again.

Many students actually find it flattering to be told things
they already know from school, provided it's not the entire
course, and provided the information is put over tactfully.
Maybe you should acquire their sixth form syllabus and see
what they were taught at school, remembering that if it says
'proteins' it does not mean they can sketch a haemoglobin
molecule. Even if your topics overlap with those of other
university courses, leave them in if the reports trickling
through on these lectures are unfavourable. It is strange
though how little co-operation there is between academics
when it comes to dovetailing courses, but perhaps we are
too individualistic a race. If only we didn't have to wait
twenty years to discover that the member of staff in the
laboratory next door had also spent the past twenty years
giving the self-same course as us to the self-same audience
as us. 'Well, it doesn't do them any harm!'

4. Have I a convincing story to tell?

This is probably the most important question of all. Look at your headings and ask yourself what connection there is between them. Wearing my students' shoes does one topic lead naturally, even compulsively, to the next, or do I feel like yawning 'so what?' after each one? Have I a good story-line linking different groups of topics? Is there an overall plot for the term? If the answers are negative, then your lectures will be of the genre: 'That's all I want to say about atoms' – lecturer glares at the clock – all the students glare at the clock – the lecturer fumbles protractedly with his notes – 'Now I want to talk about bacteria' – general sighs and all eyes longingly return to the clock. Such lectures seem the perfect recipe for boredom; hour after hour of it, term upon term of it. Boredom calculated to drive even the most devoted from physics to astronomy, from astronomy to philosophy, from philosophy to psychology, and so to the Health Centre. Indeed, the single word 'boring' is probably used more often than any other in describing courses. If we have no coherent line of thought at this stage, it will be hard to avoid the criticism later. It really is surprising how little we pick up from the theatre or novels. Any clergyman speaking on 'three points' may get laughed at by his congregation, yet there may be more connection between his three topics than between *any* three of ours. A rather amusing game to play solo is to get hold of a colleague's course outline and try to imagine how he connects together his topics; topics which read like: 'Newton's equations, rolling down an incline, denaturation of proteins, the philosophy of science'. Makes you wonder what the philosophy is going to be like.

We should now have a reasonable number of headings down on paper. We can see how one leads to the next, how the plot thickens. We can see how the interest will be maintained by not dilly-dallying on too many corollaries, which tend to be action-halters anyway. We have made sure that we will not be developing major new techniques which we then fail to apply, and that we will not have to side-track later to cover ground that should have been covered earlier. We may even have built in topics which can safely be ignored if, as is likely, we have still over-estimated the amount of material which can be covered.

Of course, many a good set of lectures has been written which did not start life on such a framework. The chances are, however, that if we beginners omit this stage and just start writing as the spirit moves us, not only will we lack any overall purpose, but we will spend a disproportionate time on what should be preliminaries. The core will be non-existent. You and I may also find that we simply haven't got time to get the detailed notes in order before term begins. If this possibility becomes a reality, then at least we will have something to meander along. In addition it is no harm to publish this framework abroad so that, quite apart from detailed criticisms, any major misemphasis can be spotted and corrected at this stage.

CHAPTER

3

Lecture writing

As it stands, the framework which we have evolved for the course is pretty dry. It's the sort of ordered outline that might equally well have served as the skeleton of a book. But a lecture must be no recital of one's *magnum opus*. If it is, government economists may justifiably contrast the cost of a student at university with one taking a correspondence course and come to embarrassing conclusions. No, in current jargon, we must not enter a lecture theatre to recite, or to teach – that is much too paternalistic – we must go in and create 'learning situations'. It means giving the kids mud and letting them discover what to do with it. On the arts side, one gathers that lecturers should ooze inspiration, omitting the facts altogether, while we on the science side, with many necessary facts of life to implant, must be careful to sugar the pill. We are to be part instructional, part inspirational. Making no bones about my own paternalistic style, here are some questions to keep in mind as you set to work injecting inspiration and instruction into your titles.

1. How sophisticated should I be?

Using the same set of headings we might be able to prepare one course of lectures that would go down well at a research scientists' meeting and another that would win rounds of applause at a mothers' meeting. Our strongest temptation will be to play to the academic élite. The élite of the class, those who will proceed to research, must be impressed at any cost. We will dot every *i*, cross every *t*, so that when these students graduate they will choose us for their research supervisor. Good research students produce many papers, and many papers is what promotion committees like. As for the rest of the class, we won't need them to remember our names. They will unfortunately: they will plague us for references in the years to come, but these requests will be summarily dealt with. Industry for them.

Students themselves may lead you into overpitching. To demonstrate their cleverness, the brighter ones will swot up the most obscure information and then put you through a stiff general knowledge quiz at the end of a lecture. You will mumble something about having another lecture to give but promise to take up their points next week. Which you do; only you go one better by devoting a whole lecture to answering the query about why the acetylcholine content is $350\mu g/gm$ Wet Weight in an octopus's brain, but only 2.6 in a dog's brain. You must also be on your guard against the well-scrubbed student who asks, pleadingly, why you don't use 'generalised relativistic quantum-mechanical coordinates' in discussing flagella. Resist the temptation to comply; instead ask him if he knows why $v = u + at$. With all this in progress, it may be difficult to fathom that the majority of the class are at sea, and have been since the first lecture. Indeed you wil not wish to know they are lost if you retain your own undergraduate-day attitudes towards the less gifted; the ones who thought that the indicator went in the burette and that cot was the integral of tan.

Now is the time for us to sink our modesty and declare that truthfully we are, and always have been, a cut above the others. With our first class degrees we are in the top ten per cent. The bulk of our class will, however, obtain lower second or third class degrees. We will therefore try and employ the sort of argument that will be appreciated by the lower second class students; and it will be difficult for us to understand how their minds operate. How's that for condescension? Occasionally we will introduce something stronger, if only to pacify those who claim to have 'heard it all before', though these claimants become more muted once the examination results are published, and occasionally we will be very naïve indeed to give some encouragement to the floundering. This might lead us, for example, in one and the same lecture, to 'remember' some bizarre convergence test and to multiply out $(x - a)^2$. As beginners, we will probably remember too many convergence tests and forget that evaluating $(x - a)^2$ is difficult. We will demonstrate too many ways of tackling a problem, describe too many pieces of apparatus, insert too many 'ifs' and 'buts', forgetting that appreciation of breadth is largely a retrospective quality. We may flit through half-a-dozen different ways of making benzene from methane, thinking we are putting over beautiful examples of reaction mechanisms, but to the audience we are simply a heavily-disguised chef preparing a six-course dinner. We decide they should know that von Wilstein's doubts grow daily on the premises of statistical mechanics, but we are bewildered by the class's reluctance to calculate the probability that two of them have birthdays on the same day. We offer them twenty different methods of measuring g in the hope that one will stick, then gasp at the unchristian names they call Newton. No, having chosen the right level of sophistication, you must not spread your net too widely.

2. What attitudes will they acquire?

You might presume that we, who pass our days probing around in research laboratories asking penetrating questions, would have our class examining the foundations the minute we walk through the door. Not a bit of it. Outside the theatre we are the perfect agnostic, but once inside all we manage is 'I found it on Mount Sinai'. We can spend an entire term dishing out 'Mutagenic Agents' and produce only a flock of parrots. We can cover blackboard after blackboard with electronic wizardry and cause not a twinge of wonder. We encourage no one to be critical, let alone original. No, I am not trying to suggest that we sire Galileos in every lecture course, but that some of our powers of perception, our open-mindedness, our originality and our humility, might occasionally be rubbed into the class. However, let us sow our virtues sparingly, not all in any one course, emphatically not all in a single lecture. As the more traditional are quick to point out, society will not thank us for engineers who, on being asked to build a bridge, sit in contemplation on the banks of the river, watching the rest of humanity as they paddle their canoes. There are more than enough mechanical skills to be required in three years as it is. There is enough questioning abroad without us stirring the waters further, thank you very much.

This questioning attitude will be nothing new to many of our students. Thanks to such schemes as the Nuffield Foundation Science Teaching Project, for example, dogmatism has been put out the back door and has been replaced by find-it-out-for-yourself and by an awareness of tautology. Things have changed since we were at school! Unaware of this shift in emphasis, you may drop such clangers as stating that objects fall because of gravity, that wires snap when the applied stress exceeds the breaking stress, and that catalysts act by speeding reactions. Drop these and they won't love you any more. Nor will they appreciate dozens of methods of measuring every quantity you mention. They will be much more querying than you were as first-year students and you will be expected to come clean about the models you are employing.

Now all of this can introduce very real problems if you have been told to prepare a course of lectures on 'The Growth Media for *E. coli* Bacteria', but lack the courage to ask the professor how he can possibly justify such a course; even why he is holding on to his chair. Surely the place for fifty-odd growth media is the textbook, or rather the handbook? Yes, indeed it is if your only idea is to get hold of the handbook and copy it out. As an alternative, try embracing the much-maligned historical approach. Try tracking down the original research papers for clues as to why one brew was superseded by another and how it affected the bugs; there must be some reason for a change even if it is only financial. You may decide to add authority to your lectures by quoting from these papers; worth while provided the papers have some life to them and not just the usual collections of clichés. Such publications are, of course, hard to come by. Better still, try and search out some rather savoury correspondence on the media. (Even fake it?) That should spice things up a bit. Almost any device to avoid the 'That was the twenty-seventh medium. Here is the twenty-eighth' approach; the approach which poisons student relations with *E. coli*, bacteriology, and ultimately with biology. Besides humanising a very impersonal subject, this technique should give the class some insight into scientific methodology. And your concern, to use the word in its old nonconformist sense, will become theirs.

When all is said and done, the psychologists say, it's our attitude towards the subject, rather than the syllabus content, which determines the student's reaction to our course. Our whole approach should be infective. If the subject bores us, it will assuredly bore the class. If it excites us it may, but only may, excite them. If we are critical they will become critical. If we extrapolate, they will extrapolate. However, we must not rush into self-congratulation when several of our students win Nobel Prizes. These ones may have been so highly motivated that even our worst efforts failed to put them off the scent. Perhaps, more than we care to realise, our most telling successes are our failures.

3. What terminology should I employ?

To us *F* is for fluorine. To our flock, who also have lectures from Tom, Dick and Harry, *F* is for fluorine, Farad, Helmholtz free energy, Gibbs free energy, filial generations, and the sixth corner of an octagon. We will not know of these added complications until, marking the Christmas examination, we discover some lamb who is under the impression that space is filled with regular octohedra, designed by Gibbs (but maybe it was Helmholtz's son) and that it is morally wrong to destroy our sacred heritage by 'fluorodinidating' the water supplies, etc. Hopefully, none of us will ever fully understand how such impressions are gained, yet all of us should consider to what extent we will employ internationally agreed nomenclature, and how far we should go it alone. We may decide to go it alone in 'subsidiary' courses when the subject is not developed to the point where subscripts and superscripts become a positive blessing. At elementary levels, F_{ij}^{k} may be read as some ogre, while attempts at copying down an $\mathscr{H}$ will resemble Harris's attempts at negotiating Hampton Court Maze. As to units, find some other excuse for not adopting SI than the overworked one that so long as *The Java Journal of Palaeontology* accepts papers in imperial yards, even so long must our students use imperial yards. For imperial yards read c.g.s. units.

With the contents, the level to be aimed at, and the approach, settled, detailed preparation of your notes can begin. All those texts you read while brooding over what topics to include should now be discarded and you should sit down with only a blank pad and the lecture outline before you. Drastic action maybe, but it will guarantee a personal flavour to your words, go a long way to ensuring that the story line is being held, and will help maintain a uniform level of sophistication. As you write you will find yourself devising arguments to be found in no textbook, ones which may be a distinct improvement. You may even hear yourself deliver the lecture, watch yourself write on the board, and sense the audience's reaction. Be less courageous, sit with texts A, B and C, and your lectures will be a mixture of the styles of A, B and C. Not only will the level of argument fluctuate erratically, but you will be emotionally detached from what story there is. You will be discouraged from getting to grips with the subject, and encouraged to copy out blindly. And if you intend to copy out arguments mechanically, why not give them the page numbers and let the class copy them out for themselves? You say they can't because A and B are out of print, and C isn't in the college library. Then, hang the copyright laws, have them stencilled. Small wonder students so often state they would rather have stencilled hand-outs than lectures; at best they often find it hard to spot the difference. There is, of course, a legitimate place for the occasional hand-out containing, e.g. numerical tables, detailed drawings, or book lists. They are also useful for presenting alternative arguments, such as the sophisticated ones we ruled out because only ten per cent of the class would have understood them. When more than occasional, these handouts remain unread.

There is one, and only one, area of lecturing techniques where advice is always available; the pure mechanics of writing down notes. Everyone who has ever spoken in public will clamour to offer advice. On the one hand you will be told that a leather-bound postcard-size ring folder is vital for success, and on the other that loose sheets of foolscap are necessary to get the whole of a proof on one page. Someone may even suggest that, like him, we should never use notes. No need to in these elementary classes, you can always ask them what you did in the last lecture. (Whatever did he get his lectureship for?) And everyone, from the professor to the vicar, will admonish you on the need to underline salient points; not even the colour of the ink will be left to chance.

Joking apart, the sheer mechanics are worth considering briefly. On the question of paper, separate sheets in a folder are often preferable to a notebook, in spite of the odd missing page. The notebook smells of permanence and won't encourage you to alter things next year, still less in twenty years' time. Small sheets, or cards, will tempt you to write small, and later on to hold them six inches from your eyes. The proper place for notes is several feet away, so write an appropriate size. Then should you not write out precisely what is to go on the board, even what should be underlined? If you don't, nervousness will probably drive you to put up trivialities which the class will, not unnaturally, think are significant. How about employing some consistent system for numbering equations and paragraph headings? Without this, you may find yourself having to refer back to 'the equation which was about here in the last lecture, the one with the $sin^4(x/2)$ in it'.

Your greatest failing in preparing lecture notes may be to put down too much on paper. You probably have no intention, indeed you should have no intention, of delivering a eulogy to some Eastern potentate. Therefore no purpose is served by writing down every word or every punctuation mark which takes your fancy. What is useful are a few key words to remind you of salient points. It is also worth while scattering instructions among equations on how to go from one line to the next, e.g. 'Divide across by 2'. It may be obvious to the class, but it will not be obvious to a very flustered you. As these reminders must be found during a few quick downward glances, I personally write them in red ink. In addition, I write what is to go on the board in black, keep blue for jokes and reserve green for hints on demonstrations.

How long does it all take? Believe it or not, it is not unusual to find a *conscientious* teacher spending at least twenty hours in preparing a one-hour lecture, and up to forty hours is not unheard of. With the term's notes completed, a useful final exercise is to divide the total number of pages by the total number of lectures. Chew you answer over and take appropriate action.

It is now October.

CHAPTER

4

The world première

There are several hundred freshers inside. I know this because I can see them through the gap between the doors. They are inside and I am outside. Very shortly I am going to have to open those doors and set off for the lecture bench. Now the bench is a long way off and there is a lot of empty space between me and that bench; wide open space where I will be exposed to view. Can I make the journey quickly enough? Or will I trip up and fall? And if this happens should I crawl backwards out the door, or should I keep crawling forwards and hide behind the bench? The class might then mistake me for an imbecile and excuse me from lecturing.

The last occasion I spoke in public was some twenty years ago. It was at my primary school's Christmas concert that I, the Hamlet of the class, was firmly planted on a wobbly platform, and told to soliloquize to the world on my aspirations, thus:

> 'I wish I were a traffic light,
> To make the traffic stop.
> > (A lot of hand-waving.)
>
> I wish I were traffic light,
> To make the traffic go.'
> > (Even more hand-waving.)

Would that these sentiments were mine today. I was told then that every word of mine had been clearly heard, and that my every gesture had been understood. Even the uncle and aunt who sat in the back row but two, where the seats were cheapest, said they had missed nothing and that they were sure the West End could not contain my equal. Whatever has become of all that youthful confidence? I was led to believe it increased with age, but, instead of crystallising out, it has evaporated.

Alan Walton, why did you turn down that research post with The Association of Deep-Sea Trawler Owners? It's true that the salary offered was lower than your present one, but not that much lower when you consider the income-tax. Answer this: which deep-sea trawler research officer is presently standing outside a lecture theatre nervously waiting to walk in? How tranquil life must be out there far away from humanity with the waves lapping against the hull and the moon shimmering across the waters. Down below the tars are now being lulled to sleep with a mermaid's song, knowing that the great, still stars keep their silent watch atop. And when the gentle hand of dawn is stretched forth across the seas, and Pliedes puts out her lamp, they will awaken fresh with the tang of salt in their nostrils.

Reflections in bad prose will get you nowhere. Open that theatre door and get inside.

You have very probably been savouring your first words for some weeks now. There is every chance that you will have learnt them word perfect. A word of advice: don't utter a single syllable of them. If you had planned to say, for example: 'This course of sixteen lectures will deal with the structure of the cell nucleus, its enzyme systems and with the role of cytoplasmic bodies', and you try to, it will be the last thing you will say. Although you will be unaware of the fact you will have succeeded in giving your audience the impression that there are to be sixty lectures, that you are going to talk about nuclear strictures, and that in your considered opinion the nucleus surrounds the cytoplasm. You will appreciate neither the hearty laughter nor the clapping. Even if you do hit it off it will read like a papal encyclical and they will start to wonder who you are, and what you could possibly know about it. Quite the wrong approach. Pause and think.

What, more than anything else, do you wish for at this moment? Why, that the floor will dissolve away beneath you or, failing this, that you will stop quaking and start to do yourself justice. In short, you wish to be your own sweet simple self.

The impression that you are Minerva with trousers on can be delayed till later in the term, but action cannot. As a means of inducing self-confidence, the pre-planned joke can be dismissed since you will forget the funny line or, if you remember the funny line, you will forget the bit that went before, without which the funny line isn't funny. Instead try telling them your name, if you can recall it. Fail to disclose this information and you will be rechristened 'the short chap with glasses, the one who's bald, in his late forties'. Even tell them that you are as raw to the game as they are; but don't expect to get any sympathy on this score. Then read out appropriate, or inappropriate, paragraphs from your favourite text on lecturing techniques – anything to break the ice. Try the effect of chatting to them over a cup of tea about what life was like here long ago, in the far off pioneering days when the university was all wooden huts and seas of mud. 'The huts had springy floors, so we knew when someone was coming along the corridor. The mud was slippery and oozed everywhere. You couldn't walk, we had to shuffle. There were only twenty-three people in the entire university then. We addressed the vice-chancellor by his Christian name, and he addressed the porter by his. There only was one porter, and he was part-time. In between spells of duty he would make our mid-morning coffee and our afternoon tea, which we had together in a big room at the end of a hut. At other times this room was used for lectures. Where we are now, a poultry farm once stood. The farmer who owned it was a 'nut' with all sorts of crackpot ideas on what food was good for chickens. The chickens didn't like the food. Then, one day they rose up and, having pecked his eyes out, they killed that farmer and feasted on his innards. He is scarcely remembered now and chickens continue to be fed on oats.' And old yarn you care to concoct will do. It is quite irrelevant that you only arrived here five days ago and that five minutes ago you had to ask someone the way to this theatre.

Whatever steps you take to induce the feeling of confident authority there is one golden rule that must be observed throughout: *Look them in the face.* Appreciate that there actually is a class before you; one composed of real live chicks. Look at all sections of the class. Even pick out random individuals in different parts of the room and stare their eyes out. Talk yourself into believing that these are no stuffed birds. That one. could she have been headgirl? He looks like a drug addict and I am sure that those two do everything the Sunday papers say they all do. Which of them, I wonder, will fail their exam next year, and be thrown out? Which of them will fail their exam next year but be allowed to stay on because they have either lain on a psychiatrist's couch or sat on a professor's knee? The Duke's daughter is here – she deserves a particular type of grin. Now try and imagine what you would say to each if you met them socially. And if, after all this, you still cannot raise a smile, then adopt Dr Kitson Clark's suggestion and repeat 'What a crew!' to yourself. But be absolutely certain of this: unless you come to grips at this stage with the truism that you are communicating man to man, the rest of your lecturing days will be spent chatting, in a quiet unassuming manner, to the woodworm in the front bench. For all I know to the contrary, woodworm may appreciate such flattery; but your chicks won't. So, *look them in the face*, and no nonsense.

This book will have failed miserably in its intentions if you are not completely relaxed by now. Old witty you, excreting self-confidence, dribbling enthusiasm, should be raring to go. But not too fast; there are some preliminaries to canter through first. Shouldn't you, for example, give the class some picture of what the course is about? This will, necessarily, be vague (they haven't taken it yet) and, mercifully, will not consist of choice readings from the university prospectus. However, if your course-outline has not merited a place in this publication, no harm is done in having it prepared as a lecture hand-out. Before many lectures are over, the class will be eager to learn which ditch is coming up next. On the question of hand-outs, if these are left on the benches before the lecture begins, you will be saved the acute embarrassment of having nothing to say while they are being slung around or, alternatively, of saying everything before they are in anyone's hands.

To keep on friendly terms with 'educational technologists', you should also distribute copies of your 'Course Objectives' – in plain English, how you expect the students to have changed after they have taken the course. To prepare objectives, put down in writing your thinking behind the course. If you will expect them to reproduce the line-by-line steps in deriving $E = mc^2$ then say so. If you will only expect them to be able to quote the result, say so. If you are only deriving $E = mc^2$ to show how a scientist operates, and will only expect them to write an essay on 'the scientific method', spell this out. In the good old days, when students were students, they deduced all this from examination papers! Nowadays we give them a sheet of paper stating: 'When you have completed this course you should be able to: (1) Given an unlabelled diagram, assign names and functional descriptions to the main parts of the human eye. (2) Name three examples of sensory receptors becoming fatigued by prolonged stimulation and describe the effects produced by such fatigue. (3) Illustrate in at least three separate contexts, the reciprocal interaction of science and technology by interrelating correctly groups of concepts, discoveries and technological achievements, producing your own examples . . .'! Still, I suppose ticking off a list as term proceeds does induce a sense of achievement.

Next you will want to say something about appropriate textbooks. Here I have my own student memories of vast lists of out-of-date, out-of-print, books being laboriously chalked up. First an author's name, any author's name, was written up. If the name was Brown or Smith the initials were kept a dark secret, but when it was Zuckermann we learnt of all the vicar's names for him. Then followed a title, any titles. Had the work in question been called *Tertiary Amines* we would hear it as *Organic Chemistry*. They were all *Organic Chemistry* if carbon got a mention in these texts, and were all *Atomic Physics* if the authors had out-lived Dalton. Then there were the lecturers who gingerly carried in a dozen ill-assorted books with blue and green covers and told us that 'these are them'; nothing more. What we had hoped for, of course, was a few well-chosen titles with a few succinct words on each, including the names of any sources tapped by the lecturer.

Text for first-year courses must be chosen with particular care; remember the great stampede to buy whatever was recommended in your first lecture at university? Publishers know of this impulse in freshers and attempt to seduce us into recommending an unlikely, ill-selling, text by the lure of a complimentary copy. For our part we have succeeded in seducing five guineas (£5.25) books out of publishers on the pretence that we intend adopting them as first-year texts. Better keep to your word. The publishers will have talked all the local bookshop managers into stocking up with hundreds of copies of the work. You will not be very popular with these managers when the expected stampede fails to materialise.

This is also the hour to say 'a word or two' on your style of lecturing. For example: 'I have so planned things that even if you only copy down what is on the board you will at least have got the major points. You should therefore assume, albeit tentatively, that what is on the board has some intrinsic value. I would also suggest that you should preserve for posterity some of the gems dropping from my lips –

I was going to say pearls thrown to the swine.' All good donnish jokes, which will be wasted on them. If you intend using a system of numbered headings, now is also the time to break the news, quoting §4.9.17(b) as an example.

Your first lecture may not be the most appropriate occasion, but you should be quick to lay your cards on the table. If you are, say, a chemist or biologist who adopts an empirical approach to problems then make this fact plain to the class. If you are the sort of mathematician or physicist who makes sure that all your i's are dotted, spell out your approach. If order-of-magnitude answers satisfy you, again state this plainly. Unless we all lay our cards on the table, students will somehow acquire the notion, probably from their hardest-selling lecturer, that there is but one true scientific method and that all others are therefore heretical. Mathematics majors will have no conception how physicists can be so casual about formulating problems, while chemists will be exasperated by the failure of biochemists to discuss reaction mechanisms. Five minutes spent describing how you approach problems in your discipline will be five minutes well spent. Even contrast your techniques with those of your colleagues, who, remember, will also be lecturing to the class. Until we all declare our hands, students will continue to dismiss chemists who cannot, or do not, solve differential equations, and physicists who know that a potassium permanganate solution cleans glass but have no idea why.

Since the students are as untrained at their end of things as we are at ours, offer them suggestions about note-taking. Point out the advantages of taking notes down in rough first, to be rewritten in their own words as soon as possible afterwards. Let them know there will be fewer worked examples than at school, so they should devote some time to problem-solving. If these rather obvious truths remain unsaid they will remain unthought of; until finals when half the class will discover that they took not a single note during the previous three years. Then these dear permissive students will complain that someone should have told them to. How were they to know? It's us who are responsible for their 'thirds'.

This little speech will have occupied the first five to ten minutes and will have given you an easy let-in to your coming-out lecture. Like the succeeding few lectures, you should have planned this one to be relatively elementary, content-wise. In it you may only 'remind' them of what they already know, possibly employing a new, more personal, viewpoint. Not only will this allow the freshman to re-establish his self-confidence within his new surroundings, but it may also take care of the fact that you are probably over-pitching anyway. Of course, if the approach and content are identical to the ones he met at school you will be thought of as condescending and this will, naturally, be resented. It is, perhaps, consoling that even the most sophisticated student will often fail to see through such crude ploys as 'reminding'.

Technique-wise your first lecture should also be as simple as possible. You will have a tough enough time just keeping in touch with your audience; so keep the 'distractions' to a minimum. For the time being, shun complex demonstrations, projectors, TV gear, and all the other paraphernalia of educational technology. Attempt a complex demonstration if you must but, be forewarned, it won't work. Why? Because you will forget to switch on the mains. You won't notice your mistake but the audience will. What happens now is that, instead of stating quite frankly that you have no idea what is wrong (someone in the audience will tell you) you start mumbling excuses. You suggest 'It must be the weather' and the audience giggle. You start to sweat. 'Well then, a fly got in the works' and the giggles turn to laughs. You decide your theories will carry more conviction if made quantitative: 'The damp weather has probably caused a resistor to discharge'; a plausible enough excuse were we not experiencing the longest drought on record. The audience burst into unmingled joy, so you next try laying the blame fairly and squarely on the shoulders of that miserable fly. 'The fly has probably got jammed between the grid and the anode.' Then it happens; the door bursts open and in walks the Duke to see what the uproar is all about. The general tenor of the audience's remarks is that they would rather have lectures from His Grace than you.

There are two nettles to be grasped from your very first lecture; facing up to the audience and writing on the board. Perhaps enough has already been said on the first of these; as to the blackboard, it is so vital a tool for the scientist that a later chapter will be devoted to its headaches. But here and now we should examine the temptations awaiting us as we come and go from talk to chalk. An example will help.

The lecture is on 'Gas Models', a heading that went up at the beginning. Using our hands we describe the erratic behaviour of a smoke particle in air; we note the audience reaction to semaphore instruction. We introduce the words 'Brownian Motion', pick up a piece of chalk, write up this pre-planned heading, and return to face the class. Involved again: 'I wonder why this is? Any ideas? Is that the only possible explanation?' Maybe these are rhetorical questions which we soliloquise over. We can spot the important cues with a few quick downward glances at our notes, lying there on the bench. But now we wish to discuss the mechanism in a highly quantitative manner, and we require information on those pages. This is where many go wrong, wilfully wrong. They pick up their notes and regress to the board. Their notes are six inches from their eyes, their back is to the class. Never again will their faces be seen by man. This is just about the greatest pitfall there is in lecturing and the hardest to get out of. You will avoid falling into the trap if you leave your notes on the bench and rely on your short-term memory for the journey to the board. That's right; you will regularly have to return to the bench and so face the class. And by 'face' I mean 'face', full-face. Without notes at hand you will also have to cogitate on how to go from one line to the next. This, in turn, will add a sense of urgency to your delivery. And if your subject is so precious that you feel, on principle, the notes must not leave your hands, do sprinkle instructions like 'look at class', 'return to bench', and 'did they understand that?' among the equations. Then obey these instructions to the last tittle.

Some months ago we planned precisely what was to go on the blackboard. We have rigidly adhered to this plan of writing up everything we thought out in advance, and nothing that was unpremeditated. But suppose we had never signed the pledge, what would we be up to in this, our first lecture? Why, we would be making occasional disturbed sallies to the board to write up the most trivial of information, which would then be given undue weight by the audience. Instead of the emphasis we had intended, the notes taken from the board would have read '1827, movement, Brown, bombardment, 6×10^{23}'. What's all this about then? An account of the Napoleonic wars?

Time flies. We sneak a glimpse at our watches rather than look directly at the clock, for this could only give the class our ideas. There are five minutes left. Should we start a new topic? Never. We would lose all composure as the seconds run past. We would break all the rules, get into a ruffle, and become the naked ape we were one long hour ago. Let us therefore wrap up decently what we have just unbosomed. Perhaps we could give them some clues about our next lecture, leaving them with a cliff-hanger.

We gather up our notes, clip them together, and walk out. We feel physically shattered. Does everyone have this feeling after a lecture? Yes; I should have taken that job at sea.

CHAPTER

5

On stage

As soon as my first lecture was over, I slunk out of the nearest door and escaped. As fast as my legs would carry me I escaped to the seclusion of the office. I could hear the growing murmurs of discontent, the steps coming ever closer. But I had made it. I locked the door and deliberated on what action to take when the knock came. Will I pretend I am not in? Will I hear them cry 'He must be in?' I looked out the window and gauged my height above ground. But the knock never came. And when all was still and the stars began to brighten the dark October sky, I cautiously turned the key, had second thoughts, and relocked the door. I could see them leering away outside. But it was deserted. Very quietly I slipped out through a side gate, unnoticed by even the night watchman. I was soon home and almost dry. The remaining hours of night were spent contemplating why the gods ever saw fit to bring me into this cruel, unloving, unlovely, world.

If you get these sort of feelings keep them under your hat. You would prefer to say that, perhaps, your first lecture had not gone quite as well as you might have wished, *n'est-ce pas?* Never mind, we all have these little blemishes. Before long though I will teach you how to varnish them over. But first we must bolster up your self-confidence.

Just think of it, your show is good for an eight week run with a guaranteed audience of several hundred. Any West End actor worthy of the name would jump at the opportunity of such a season. And you are unenthusiastic. Your theatre has no cramping proscenium arch. It has good sight-lines and is of intimate size. And you have a one-man show into the bargain.

The more perceptive you are the more likely are you to suspect that I am about to exhort you to enrol at drama school. Already you can see yourself taking last long fare-wells of the homestead, of the children and of the wife. The winding road to The Royal Academy of Dramatic Art opens up before you. You can picture it all; the garret, you, your tiny frozen hands, little Mimi. Your hopes are quite un-founded. Only the elements of histrionics are required. Good techniques can make a poorly thought out course seem acceptable. Bad techniques will take the edge off a good course.

Let's attend to your voice first. As you know, the two qualities which you can most readily manipulate are pitch and intensity; the qualities which determine the impact of your words. Perhaps you think of them as independent. But are they? Try this experiment. One dark night when the sky is clear, creep out of doors. Bay softly to the moon. Now loudly to the moon. Did you notice how, as the intensity of your voice increased so did your pitch? Like a mad dog almost. While this is unlikely to disturb any who are abroad when the moon is full, it can be very tiring to an audience if the same phenomenon occurs indoors. Fast speaking or 'nerves' may also bring about this rise in pitch. So keep a constant watch on where your pitch is straying and take deliberate steps to check it. It can be checked with deter-mination but, at least in my own experience, the fault is largely self-eliminating as we gain in confidence. Because we hold our heads up, because we look at the audience, because we sense their reactions and respond to them, we find ourselves entering into dialogue with the class rather than haranguing them. We become ourselves and speak naturally. Indeed a soft natural voice is probably more 'audible' anyway than a loud shrill one. Unless your theatre was built in Queen Victoria's hey-day, or seats five-hundred, you should not need to turn up the volume by much. If sound amplification is laid on, speak in a totally normal manner and don't swallow the microphone. This much is certain: you should never have to pose that most meaningless of questions: 'Can your hear me up the back?'

Speed and 'nerves' may not only affect your pitch but they may lead to bad breathing – so say the histrionic textbooks. Bad breathing is a euphemism for swallowing frantic gulps of air at the wrong moments. This produces great shortages of air just when you need it most. So you fade away and die in mid-sentence. A simple check well worth making is the level of your water consumption. If you cannot get through a lecture without draining the barrel dry, then you are probably using your voice incorrectly. Only curse the chalk-dust as a last resort.

In everyday conversation we continually adjust the pitch, intensity and speed of delivery to suit the mood of the occasion. We have one voice for our lawyer, another for our beloved. Our manner of speaking to an eighty-year old and to an eight-month old are quite different. We know the value of silence and when a rich booming voice can be used with effect. When excited we accelerate. When near the root of things we slow down. Such expressiveness is so natural that any who have none of it quickly earn for themselves the reputation of bores; quite irrespective of the wisdom of their words. An audience likewise finds a monotonous voice exasperating. They have to study the word context to determine the significance of what the lecture is about, and soon give up the effort. So would you if this happened in the legitimate theatre.

The easiest way of securing a natural delivery is to relax completely. Even if we cannot prevent inner tensions we should at least be able to train ourselves to sound natural. After all the professional actor does it daily when he walks on to play an assumed role. Let's look at some of his elementary techniques to see if they might not fit you. For example: at

some stage or other every actor comes forward to the foot-
lights and speaks in an almost inaudible whisper. The
audience have been taken into his confidence; again it's no
more than what happens in ordinary conversation. So the
next time you have your own highly personal doubts about
some piece of apparatus, or conceptual model, try talking
softly of them to your audience. For maximum effect walk
around to the front of the lecture bench, lean nonchalantly
on it, and chat. Chat to them about your failings, your
doubts, and the problems which lie ahead. Chat away; they
are human and love gossip. I guarantee the effect is such
that you will never again speak in a monotone. Now think
about when a declamatory style might be appropriate
Should it be employed when describing the work of some
bombastic scientist? Or should it be reserved for the arro-
gant assumptions?

Overwork these simple techniques and their effect will
soon vanish. Experiment with new ones. Discover for yourself the use that can be made of deliberate long silences, of
one word every five seconds, and of five words to the second.
Experiment with growling and with whistling. Should you
sing, exploit this talent also. If these techniques seem too
advanced then try the effect of weeping as you describe the
breakdown of classical physics. Hold back nothing as you
paint the futile attempts which were made to patch it up.
Make it seem as if classical physics was very close to your
heart. For a change, see if you can have them rolling in the
aisles as you attempt a realistic assessment of His Grace's
contribution to the subject. With luck, the Palladium will
be able to fit you in with a spot when your contract is terminated here.

Ideas such as these are apt to occur at all sorts of odd hours
of the day and night, mostly during the latter. They may
hit you as you read over your notes in advance of the lecture.
When they do so, it is well to script them since they can
easily be forgotten in the heat of the moment. If you just go
in with the vague intention of modulating your voice you

will probably end up simply emphasising every 'the', or something equally inconsequential.

The well-intentioned arts-man may advise you against so much as opening a lecture theatre door until after you have devoured Swift, Goldsmith, and all their works. Face up to these people. No half-measures about enjoying *Lilliput*, or having done *The Vicar of Wakefield* at school. Tell them you realise that the words they use are as important as the ideas they clothe. They cannot divorce one from the other. We can; although mathematical symbolism may fulfil this role for us, leaving our words to pass the time of day. Because of this they can easly become cliché-ridden. It needn't be so. Adopt a more informal style of lecturing and good plain colloquial English can result.

What perhaps worries people most of all on the speech question is 'er and 'um'ing. They fret about it if they do. If they don't, they fret about not being conscious of whether they do it or not. They think they might, but are not sure. At the risk of standing accused of letting the side down, let me state my own blunt belief that 95 per cent of 'er' and 'um'ing arises because lecturers don't know their subject. They have no idea of what they are going on about. They are so uncertain of what should come next that they have to 'er' and 'um' while they chew the cud. Their uncertainty may also be shown up in sentences left unfinished. In a way it's a good thing that it's hard to conceal our ignorance; this is hardly the object of the exercise. How dare they even attempt these confidence tricks!

Many a comedian has established his reputation by the constant repetition of certain words and phrases. The path to stardom is tougher going in the academic sphere, where audiences have been known to refer disparagingly to stock phrases. It is interesting how it is never levelled as a serious criticism against a good lecturer, but is it always pulled out of the bag if he has other more serious failings. The art probably lies in using these phrases very selectively. One we could well be without is 'doing'.

You never 'do' topics if the course has been imaginatively constructed.

Jokes are a much bigger problem altogether. In spite of a strong temptation to do otherwise, all I will say on the subject is that if they really are inextricably bound up with some vital point in the course it won't matter whether they succeed, fall flat, or even whether the whole audience collapses in laughter at you making a fool of yourself. The vital point will be remembered just because it was so inextricably bound up. If you feel that it is asking too much of anyone to concentrate for an hour on such a subject as yours, then the utterly irrelevant joke also has its place. Two small points. Should the joke be scripted, stand a minimum of twenty feet from your notes for the punch line; and if your ambition is to become a spontaneous wit, put the jokes on a three-year cycle. What can be more annoying than any joke are the 'How I won the war' stories. Remember that there are so many counter claims for having built the bomb or discovered DNA's structure that yours may be viewed with a slight degree of suspicion. Also watch those stories about having presented Medawar or Mendel with the solution to the problem; for which you received not so much as a word of mention, but which will one day all come out in the wash. They suspect this will happen. Besides they know you cannot be that old; well, not quite.

A Bath-chair is the only property you need have purchased to date. It is true that you are required to oscillate between the lecture bench and the board, but this is hardly an actor's dream of Utopia, even to one in a Bath-chair. How then should we make full use of the stage? The answer may seem obvious: put in some training for the ten-kilometre event. This is actually a perfectly acceptable solution for, as Dr G. Kitson Clark observes in his treatise *The Art of Lecturing* (Heffers, 1959), 'Some excellent lecturers I have known have travelled surprising distances.' You will have to check up on the truth, or otherwise, of the converse. There are the lecturers who amble lovingly towards the window where they quickly lose themselves through gazing rapturously at the heavens or, as is more likely in these decadent times, at some passing thing of beauty. Then there are lecturers who prefer not to wander during their lectures. They are to be seen writing pathetic little messages in the chalk-dust on the lecture bench, or curling up the corners of their notes. In their more expansive moments they will balance precariously on the edge of the raised platform or will do press-ups against the bench. Yet others of our profession go to town on the blackboard pointer. They transform it, in turn, from a billiard cue, to a bishop's crozier and then to a bean stalk. But whichever of these categories you fall into, be not faint-hearted. The audience love your little eccentricities and will never damn you for having them. Unless, that is, they occupy you to the exclusion of everything else.

We would be failing miserably if these were your only histrionic skills; admirable though they may be. Just look at the occasions when even the actor in local repertory uses the centre of the stage, and when he goes to a corner. Could you not behave like him? You hardly need be an Elizabeth Taylor or a Michael Redgrave to shrug your shoulders when you meet some anomaly; or to soliloquise off-centre as you contemplate how to slay a differential equation. Even retreating to the back of the room to 'wonder' calls for no great skills. The more ambitious of us may, however, be able to get to sleep on the bench, crawl around on the floor, or even trapeze; all to good effect. The difficulty may be not what to do, but rather how to get the self-control which stops us acting the goat unless it is one-hundred per cent in the interests of the subject. Just as in joke-telling, relevancy must be our sole criterion. But if it is genuinely relevant, the impact of you juggling with plates while cycling across a high wire will be very great.

On the question of costume, some lecturers wear gowns to keep the dust off their clothes. To others it would be a betrayal of all that was closest to their hearts – although some of these may have to watch the temptation to take on free-lance, but unpaid, modelling for Carnaby Street. There are those who see it as a sacred institution which, like the gowns, has been passed down from generation to generation, one which must on no account be slighted. 'If the institution did not have a useful function to perform it would have died out long ago. Gowns did not come about by accident; they came about by conscious design.' Indeed it must truthfully be admitted that sober black can eliminate the body and leave the audience free to concentrate on your soul. A loudspeaker approaches even closer to the ideal. Again it is argued that a gown makes each man as naked as his neighbour, so to speak. But which of us from gown-wearing universities ever attended a lecture where the gown itself was not one of the most fascinating exhibits? There were the torn ones, the ones that were once black but are now green, the ones that had seen service as blackboard dusters and are now white, and the ones which made you wonder if the wearer was legitimately qualified to do so. And the antics which could be performed with a gown. Just ask yourself whether your sports-coat has this same fascination.

Once we accept the somewhat unoriginal thesis that theatrical techniques have a valid place in the lecture theatre boundless possibilities open up. On awakening to this truth, one of my colleagues proceeded to borrow a 'bunny' from a local club. Close, but very discreet, enquiries revealed that her only role in the lecture had been to carry in a piece of apparatus; a piece of apparatus that could have been on the bench all along. This was a totally unwarranted misuse of such a lady, and contributed nothing to the class's understanding of the skeletal structure of rabbits! It was utterly irrelevant. Temptations like this may be hard to resist, but they should be very firmly nipped in the bud.

No, the sort of technique which I have in mind is the employment of several 'actors'. This can be particularly useful when, for example, we wish to query a generally held theory; a theory which we alone 'suspect'. An illustration: I have (genuinely) no faith in any textbook's explanation of surface tension but if I simply put across my own private theory the audience would have no faith in me when they stumbled upon the textbooks. Within a matter of hours there would be long queues outside the University Health Centre looking for guidance. They would complain that they had been given nothing to latch on to, that they did not know which way to turn, and that they had lost all faith in humanity. Another hour would pass and there would be a long queue outside my door; the psychiatrists who merely wish to draw my attention to the potential dangers of not giving undergraduates something to cling to; dangers which have been well documented. I would be cajoled into making a lengthy retraction in my next lecture; my unorthodoxy would be at an end. This approach would have invited disaster. So instead of hanging out my washing single-handed, a second member of faculty was brought in to assist. He was to be the straight man, the pure academic, who would present the standard textbook theory while I, the village idiot pure and simple, would make embarrassing noises and pose the sort of questions modesty prevents an audience from asking. My colleague would portray the real-life scientist; beautifully precise but rather gullible. I, the work's spanner thrower, would attempt to make the audience *think* in rather loose ways. First we each advanced our individual theories on surface tension offering them to the class and to each other. These were sales talks with no interruptions. The real fun began with each of us inspecting the other's dirty linen only to wash it publicly. The audience were drawn into the heart of the problem and were encouraged to take sides. They saw the extent to which one's personality affects even 'scientific' thinking and learnt that 'the truth' is more elusive than they had previously supposed. It may have been cheating, but the entire exercise was preplanned and the arguments deliberately kept unsophisticated enough to be understood by the first-year audience. This sort of carry on was common currency in the old days when it was known as a 'disputation'.

All the possible uses for a multiman act need not be spelt out in detail, but two or more 'lecturers' are a positive advantage if you wish to discuss relativity, to perform demonstrations, to present several techniques of differing sophistication, or merely to have someone to do the donkey-work of checking your algebra. If nothing else, sharing the stage with a second lecturer keeps you on your toes and the class on the edges of their seats. The subject becomes human and you may be able to bask in the glory of being recognised on buses in the remoter areas of the town. Much, naturally, depends on the personalities involved, but several interesting combinations could probably be found in every university department.

Needless to say, these types of techniques may not be to everyone's liking. If only because less 'ground' can be covered they will certainly not appeal to our Mr Gradgrinds. They may also over-appeal to those of us who would minimise the discipline of education.

Back to less controversial matters.

CHAPTER

6

The blackboard

Dr Kitson Clark, writing on the use of the blackboard, asserts that in his opinion 'some of the worst crimes are committed in its neighbourhood'. Several of these we have already met. Crimes such as using the board for trivialities, not using it for what is important, and whispering to it the secrets of the course. We have seen that prevention lies in planning precisely what has to go on the board, in religiously adhering to this plan (at least in the early days) and in keeping our notes firmly glued to the lecture bench. Now we must dip into the venial sins.

When we write on a board we do so on something which is a hundred to a thousand times larger in area than anything we have ever written on before, is vertical, and requires a new writing implement. So we may expect to find the same sort of mistakes as might have occurred had a painter of miniatures been commissioned to decorate the Sistine Chapel. Apart from too small detail, the perspective could have been at fault, and even the colours out of place.

As practical scientists with Ph.D.s behind us, it should be within our capabilities to work out just what size writing is required for it to be read from the back row of the theatre. Let's try. We know that when we read a book with print size of about $\frac{1}{8}$ in. we hold it around 1 ft. away from our eyes. So in a theatre where the back row is, e.g. 50 ft. away (measure it if necessary), we shall have to write in characters ($50 \times \frac{1}{8}$ in.), or about 6 in. high, for them to be clearly readable from the back. As we say in the profession: simple isn't it? Now try and write something in letters 6 in. high and see if it's quite so simple. Notice how you rely on elbow and shoulder movements and how unimportant are wrist and finger movements. So a brand new technique must be mastered, and one not made any easier by having the board vertical. It may even be desirable to creep into the lecture theatre at the dead of night and put in some practice. Should you do so, remember to try reading the board from the back row. It is no harm to occasionally leave the lecture theatre by a rear door anyway, so as to keep an eye on your handi-work. Whether you put this practice in or not, the faces of the audience will warn you when they experience difficulties with your writing. You will be able to deduce whether it is due to illegibility, to too small characters, or to both. (Work out how!) Never should you have to ask the audience can they decipher what you have just written. Of course, abso-lutely nothing will be obvious to you if you are busy natter-ing to those woodworm. I once attended a lecture-course where the entire back rows regularly brought in binoculars, but the lecturer either failed to notice this or else fell down in its interpretation. Perhaps it is relevant that he responded similarly towards a cuckoo-clock; introduced after he per-sistently overstayed his welcome.

Our sense of perspective is bound to suffer simply be-cause we have to write large while standing only a short distance from the board. Three-dimensional drawings will frequently look like something from a medieval woodcut. No doubt if we theorised long enough on the problem we would come up with a practical method of compensating for this tendency. It is not worth the labour since the neces-sary correction soon becomes second-nature, but should it fail to, be comforted that bad perspective seldom floors an audience. Why is it that so many lecturers become suicidal when they cannot draw a cube correctly while remaining oblivious of being the embodiment of every other fault in the book? Instead of informing the class what they are trying to draw, and allowing them half the time to draw one for themselves, they launch into a long discourse on the psychology and physiology of perspective. They confess to being uncertain whether their drawing is outside-in or inside-out. They remind the audience of those pictures of optical illusions which they must have seen as children. Then they pick up a cube and try to identify which corner of the model corresponds with which one on the board. This is without success, so they colour some edges of the model yellow, and some purple. The principle behind this little exercise is that, in theory, certain lines on the board can now be coloured yellow, and certain others purple. But the wished for one-to-one correspondence between the purple on the model and the purple on the drawing somehow eludes them. There is no end to it. It goes on and on and on as new techniques are brought to bear. The audience laps up every second of it: long may he continue. But he sniffs the bitter smell of defeat in his nostrils and anounces that he will return to the fray in the next lecture. Sitting at home that evening, brooding on the events of the day, he is seized by one of those flashes of inspiration given but rarely to man. It occurs to him that the same difficulties as he encountered today may arise yet again in tomorrow's lecture. To forestall this he will tip-toe back to the lecture theatre later that evening. When all his audience were abed he did return and spent a goodly three hours putting up something which could, in truth, be mistaken for a cube when viewed from somewhere. To crown his success he put in little red and yellow blobs in all the wrong corners, and then in all the right corners. This had the singular effect of converting the cube to a crystal of sodium chloride, as the legend made clear. Underneath he wrote $a = 2.81$ A and put a on his cube. Then he equated a little red blob with Na, a little yellow one with Cl, and wondered whether he had got them the wrong way around. A close scrutiny of the textbook in his hand revealed that he had not. He thought that while he was about it, he would save time tomorrow by putting up tonight his table listing all the known properties of NaCl. So everything from its cost in $ per pound to its density in gm/ml was duly written up. The task accomplished, he twirled the board around and retired for the night. The air of confidence with which he entered the room on the morrow came as a distinct surprise to the class, which, to a man, had passed the previous evening recounting the struggles over numerous cups of Nescafé. Today they had brought many friends to witness the repeat performance. But after a few well-chosen words which reminded them that at the end of the last lecture they were doing NaCl, a proud hand reached for the board. The board revolved and the masterpiece was revealed. During the thirty seconds while the board was facing their way the audience were vaguely aware of an impressionist's study of trellised roses. Or was it something else? They never did learn the answer to their question. The lecturer had moved on to do calcium chloride which, as he remarked, had rather a more complex structure. He tendered his apologies for not having had time to put up the drawing in advance of the lecture.

We might care to ask such a lecturer a number of questions. There is one we must ask. 'Why did you not prepare copies of those complex diagrams in advance of the lecture and distribute them on the day?' Leaving aside copyright questions, an electrostatic-copier and his textbook would soon have dealt with the problem. Failing this, he could have traced out the diagrams and had them cyclostyled. It hardly needs pointing out but, had he done so, little time would have been wasted and the entire audience would have seen what he was going on about. Then some of us might feel like asking why he persisted in talking so very incoherently about a subject which is discussed so very coherently in most texts. Alas, it is one of 'those' courses and he is one of 'those' lecturers. Probably the only occasion when one is justified in writing up something in advance, which is not in a hand-out, is when the clock forces us to break off in the middle of a lengthy derivation. We can then refer back, as required, to what the audience will have already copied down in the previous lecture.

Apart from causing bad perspective, another consequence of having to stand (relatively) so close to the board is that straight lines become arcs. A linear graph can quite easily end up looking like a page from Henry Moore's sketch-book; especially if you omit to label the axes. Glued feet are the cause of this affliction. The moral, of course, is to use your legs as well as your arms to shift the chalk. You get a bit of x-movement in by walking. A goutish disposition also leads people into making very limited use of the available space: in spite of vast areas of empty board everything is cramped mercilessly into one corner. How you use such an expanse will naturally depend on the geometry of the board, but if it should be 30 ft. long by 3 ft. high you will not write in a single line from one end to the other. Instead you may choose to imagine the board as divided up into a series of panels. And if you are expected to give a course of pure mathematics lectures in a room with a traditional 3 ft. × 2 ft. easel-board, don't!

Little need be said on the subject of chalk colours except to remind ourselves how we found it difficult to distinguish dark browns, blues and purples from black; and that we possibly failed to appreciate the challenge to simulate a medley of blackboard colours with only a pen and pencil at hand. We probably also failed to appreciate squeaking chalk; a tune that can be cured by simply breaking the head off.

Most of us never consider what we should be talking about while we write on the board, even if, as in mathematics, we have an immense amount of board material. There are several traditional solutions to this problem but all of these are rather unsatisfactory. The first is to shut up entirely; let only the tap-tapping of the chalk and the occasional shoo-shooing of the duster break the silence. How did this technique manage to survive the introduction of the printed word? Why were any remaining footholds not exterminated by the birth of the silent film? At the other extremity are those who are convinced that their mission in life is to get through as much material as they possibly can. Now they are intelligent enough to realise that they are endowed with lips that talk and hands that move – so why not allow the chalk to deal with one topic while the lips attend to another? A very laudable appraisal. Therefore they will talk about something new while their hands write up something which is distinctly old-hat. By this means their audience get good value for money as they hear one lecture on DNA and watch another on onions. Those who employ this technique should try watching *The Marx Brothers go West* on television to the accompaniment of a radio talk on 'The Democratic Party Convention'. Then, in between these extremities, come the good solid lecturers who will tell you what every grain of chalk-dust represents. If they write $P = \frac{1}{3} mn\bar{c}^2$ they will say 'pee equals a third em en cee squared bar'. When they write $PV = RT$ we hear 'peevy equals arty'. It's all so dull and, if the writing is as legible as it should be, quite unnecessary.

Let us try something different, taking $P = \frac{1}{3} mn\bar{c}^2$ as our example. To have reached this stage will have taken a good five minutes; a long time has therefore elapsed since the audience were first introduced to 'em', 'en' and 'cee'. By now they will have completely forgotten who, or what, they represent. Repeating *'em'*, *'en'*, and *'cee'* is no help! But they can be reminded if, as you write $P = \frac{1}{3} mn\bar{c}^2$, you say: 'So the pressure in a gas is a third the product of the mass of a molecule, times the number per unit volume, times the average value of the squares of the molecular velocities'. A great many other reminders could have been given; such as where the third came from, why the velocity occurs squared, and why the mass does not occur squared. These same type of reminders could have been introduced all along the route. Alternatively you could perhaps have told them some historical anecdote; the sort of information which is of no value to remember. What is really wanted is something along the lines of a good television commentary, but this is not an easy technique to master since our hands tend to follow our mouths, and vice-versa. What probably would have happened if you had tried to tell them, while writing $P\delta t = \frac{1}{6} nc\delta t \times 2mn$, that Boyle was an Irishman is that you would have written $B\delta I = \frac{1}{6} rs\delta h \times man$. Even silence would have been preferable to this. It can take quite some training to become so disorganised that our hands fail to follow our mouths. But those who reach this state of nirvana may also have to take heed that they do not advance to the realms of Fermi-Dirac Statistics while the audience is still befriending 'em', 'en', and 'cee'.

Whatever running commentary is adopted, most of us will find it necessary to have our backs to the class while actually writing on the board; but let us minimise the effect by turning our heads around whenever feasible. This will convince the audience that they are still very close to our hearts, and also allow us to see if they are experiencing any difficulties. The more athletic members of the profession may be able to write on the board without so much as turning a degree. Athletic or not, none of us will ever forget to leave our notes on the bench. And when you face the class, don't obscure all your wisdom by standing directly in front of what you have just written! Also, if possible, alternate the side at which you stand, both when writing and talking to minimise the annoyance to the audience in the wings.

If you want to bring out the worst in lecturers present them with a blackboard duster. The ones who are very uncertain of themselves and of their revelation will bring it into immediate use, starting with the line they have written last. In the acutely ill, the chalk is held in one hand and the duster, held in the other, is forced to follow at a distance of six inches. And if the board revolves, they can hide the skeleton even more rapidly. They soon discover that sliding panel boards can be quicker still and that, with a little ingenuity, it is possible to so use the vertical type that, as they write on an ascending board, a descending one automatically hides it all. But trying to retrieve something, hidden somewhere, can call for greater ingenuity than they possess. How Hoffnung would have loved it! Then there are those Moses-like figures who are convinced that chalk and board are the twentieth-century man's answer to lightning and tablet. Neither heaven nor hell will shift what has been revealed to them; and most certainly not a duster. So they start filling in any remaining patches of black – one word here, another there. A symbol top right, the next term, bottom left. Then they get worried that the black may be running out; they retreat several yards from the board to see if they are mistaken. Yes, they are mistaken for there is a small area just about big enough for the third term in the expression, tucked away in the top left-hand corner. The black is at last exhausted. The board, you feel, should now be ceremoniously unscrewed and presented to the nation, or auctioned at Sothebys, and that with luck it will end up deep in Texas. But these lecturers have different feelings. They can start all over again in yellow chalk. Sandwiched between these limiting forms of humanity come those who, being just a little uncertain of their revelation, decide to half obliterate it with their hands. They have another go, and then another. Trying to decipher their most recent inspiration is like trying to read a motorway sign in a snow storm.

There are other forms of visual aids besides blackboards.

CHAPTER

Screened

Michael Jones, area manager of Visual Aids Inc., mailed us a pretentious invitation some weeks ago to come along and inspect his wares. Posters are hung limply from notice-boards to remind all of the time and the place. As we glance at these mixtures of print and felt-pen, we fill with nostalgia for the days when circuses travelled our roads; they too had posters with the name of the field and the time of the show rudely inserted in some space between the clowns and the monkeys.

The show opens at 11.00 hours in the Boiler House Car Park. Mr Jones, who has likewise travelled the roads, is at home in his caravan. The caravan has ribbed aluminium steps which creak uncomfortably as we ascend. We land in plush carpet and, after exchanging our pleased to meets, are walked down both sides of the van. On Formica-topped benches proudly stand the saviours of our age. As we walk we learn how this machine has been designed specifically with Sanskrit in view and how that model over there is in daily use at The Royal College of Music, who are greatly pleased with it and have since ordered fifty more. We protest our innocence; we can neither speak one syllable of Sanskrit nor hum one bar of music. Apparently we have been mistaken for the musical Dean of Oriental Studies passing under a name which rings like ours, who once had his secretary return a business reply card expressing an enquiring interest in something or other. But this is of no consequence for such machines are equally indispensable for differential equations or fungi. We hear all their virtues, save the price, and none of their vices. After half an hour's sojourn we emerge into the sunlight clutching our expensively glossy catalogues while Mr Jones, area manager, hopes he can gladly be of future service. At 16.00 hours Mr Jones will move off to pastures new, but his place will be quickly taken by some hawker of vacuum furnaces, or ultraviolet spectrometers. Had we held the purse-strings we would have purchased the lot in the expectation that Mr Jones's firm would have responded by endowing us with a Chair. A commercially endowed Chair would leave us with more time for research than a statutory one.

One of the most persistently canvassed of visual aids is the overhead projector; which allows you to write down on a horizontal glass surface while the image is thrown over your shoulder on to a screen. Because the surface is about quarto-size and because the writing implement is a felt- or china-pen, the characters are, as claimed, often more legible than when written directly on a board. (But not when an ink pen is used – ordinary ink quickly shrinks to an invisible line in the heat.) Another allowable claim for these machines is that you can write away at high speed. And that, friends, is the core of the problem. You can indeed write very very rapidly; as any of us who have ever attended a lecture where it was used can testify. We found ourselves six lines behind the lecturer. Now six, soon it was ten, and before many minutes had passed it was not worth keeping in the race. To encourage still higher speeds, the manufacturers have conspired to design these machines to take rolls of celluloid. On these rolls the weaker brethren can, and dō, write out their entire lecture. This leaves them free to pass their hour happily breaking some handle-turning record while, puffing and panting, they mangle out the facts. The picture on the screen reminds the audience of the occasions their school's cine projector went z–z–z–z–z and the picture developed a pronounced vertical blur. At least it was switched off when this happened. As for the lecturer's commentary, it is heads faster than anything a sport's commentator could manage. Ask one of these brethren why he does it, do you know what his reply is? He does it because 'it enables me to get through so much'. You, and who else? Perhaps this strong temptation to speed could be kept under control by self-discipline. However, even if you can only slow down to a trot, there may still be a place for you and your projector in a research seminar where the audience is not expecting any notes, and where the intention is to 'run through' something which the audience can readily grasp.

On paper, overhead projectors have the real asset of forcing you to 'face' the class. However, at least in my own experience, the asset remains a paper one because the writing surface is (necessarily) so strongly illuminated that it is difficult to see the class while writing; let alone to study their reactions. You may not credit it, but some lecturers actually view this as a very enchanting facility; they can create the illusion of looking at the class without any of its attendant perils. The still weaker brethren never get round to realising that they could look up in complete safety! They lay their notes beside their machines and, without raising an eyebrow, transfer all their earthly wisdom from paper to celluloid, while the audience busy themselves in transferring it back to paper again. Some day technology will catch up with them.

To most people visual aids mean slides, and slides mean either something which takes three weeks or something which can be borrowed from the person who once gave a 'popular' public lecture (or rather who once served the public with a lecture for a consideration of twenty guineas). These are just the sort of impressions that salesman go to town on. Watch it. Unless you have your wits about you they have sold you, within ten seconds flat, the complete outfit for making slides in just so long again. Which gives you the headache of what to make slides of.

In many areas of research the photographic emulsion

occupies such a cardinal position that you would have to be blind to miss the opportunity of presenting the primary evidence when talking about these fields. Examples abound in X-ray diffraction work, in electron microscopy, in aerial surveying, and so on. Of course there are many attendant dangers; as an example will make clear. We are giving an introductory course in solid-state physics and have just completed our discussion of X-ray diffraction. Remember, the course is an introductory one. So we rightly think that we shall brighten things up by showing what actually happened when a crystal was placed between an X-ray beam and a photographic plate. The crystal, by the way, was one we had been using in our research. But instead of merely pointing out that the spots do exist and are in an ordered pattern, we wrongly decide that they must learn the whole truth. The whole truth, and shortly everything but the truth will be theirs. They will see, if they look very closely, that the spots are elliptical in shape, which probably indicates twinning. Fortunately it never enters our head to disclose what twinning is, or does. Neither are the spots of the same size, but we do remember to tell the class what determines the size of a spot. We then tell them the precise number of seconds the film was in the camera for, and the make of the developer. They learn our sorrow that the manufacturer has withdrawn the XPF 500 emulsion, and how the XPL 700F is no fit replacement. They grow wiser on the short-comings of the laboratory darkroom which are unlikely to be remedied as the professor never takes X-ray pictures. Even if the faults were put right, it still could not handle the work. And to think that all the audience wished to know was whether von Laue had been hunting for the end of the rainbow or not. And, if he failed in his search, whether it was because he had, like us, been looking at the wrong angle when he wrote $sin\ \theta = AB/BC$.

Although not a pure mathematician by training, I have every reason to believe that members of this discipline do not go on safari to hunt down axioms with a camera. This being so, it would seem to suggest that they should not, repeat not, have slide-fulls of intricate expressions. Apparently there are those, and this includes others besides mathematicians, who believe that when something is too lengthy, or too complex to be written up quickly on the board, it should be presented as a slide. And it is duly presented as a slide. A certain similarity of purpose may be noted between this response and that of the lecturer who sneaked back to draw up his cube. The traps are the same.

A much more trivial, but justified, use for the photographic emulsion is in photographing apparatus. This is not to be despised, for, occasionally, it is no harm to let the audience see the contrast between the real thing and our over-simplified diagrams. This evidence is quick to present and obviously no notes are called for. As Poo-Bah remarks, there is room for 'corroborative detail, intended to give artistic verisimilitude to an otherwise bald and unconvincing narrative'. If this detail is not provided, they may try and build a 100 GeV accelerator in the practical class when your back is turned.

Slides mean projectors, and projectors evoke in each of us many happy memories of those fumbling old fools of professors who never could put a slide into a projector the correct way up. Now, just pause and ask yourself how many ways a slide can go into a projector. And, when you have reached your answer, bitter remorse will drive you to search out the grave of he whose abilities you have spoken so lightly of. There, kneeling in the gathering dusk, you will scatter rose petals and marvel at his great skills; for, with a seven-to-one chance against him, he generally managed to get it in correctly after only five attempts. The gods may not be so kind to us, so we will mark one corner of each slide with a large white sticker. Then we shall make a special effort to remember whether the sticker should face the screen or not, and in which corner of the slide-holder the sticker should go. Now, there are in this world warped individuals who will tell stories against any lecturer who has difficulties in putting the lights out or, if he has mastered this, in putting them on again. Let them laugh. They have never seen the magnitude of the problem of trying to locate a single knob among the vast battery of switches which lurks behind every lecture bench; a battery that must make the control panels at Cape Kennedy look barren. They can laugh. With the odds so heavily against us, the surprising thing is that we only sent the blinds up and down twice; had the ventilation off and on four times; tried the 6V 120 A supply; flashed the 'Lecture in Progress' sign; and experimented with the blackboard lights. Our critics would not have narrowly escaped breaking the glass that summons the police, fire and ambulance services. And when we do eventually succeed in both darkening the room and in getting the slide in correctly, is it really so surprising that little things like removing the lens cap should be forgotten? To say nothing of the problems of locating the switch on the projector, then thinking the bulb is broken, but remembering that there is a mains switch at the other end of the lead: a lead which disappears into the thick of the audience. Nor to even begin reciting the trials of finding out how the screen is lowered and then kept from going up again. Let them try all of this and never again will they complain that the picture is out of focus, and that we haven't told them what it is of. Frankly, these are just the sort of conditions which make one forget what the picture is of, but which helps one remember that it's written on a white strip somewhere on that slide. From years of bitter experience the only advice which I would offer is that it is much better to tell them a yarn, any yarn, than risk it. If it's a linear graph it cost 100 guineas and came from Bond Street; if it's curved with dots on it the price was 1,000 guineas. And naturally we didn't ask them what they are now asking us. This is the moment when someone in the class will request that a couple of the lights be put on so that they can note down this information. Pretend you are deaf, or daft, and have been from birth. Presumably it is because the dice are so heavily loaded against the successful completion of all these operations that, should you succeed, you may feel a little proud. You have indeed every cause to be more than a little proud, but don't let your celebrations run to the limit of leaving the slide on for the next hour. The audience will be so hypnotised by the sight of a slide which is being projected the right way up on a fully-extended screen in a half-darkened room, a slide which has been talked about, that never again will they look your way. They will count one by one each glass bead; they will devour the spider who is having some difficulty deciding whether to cross the abscissa or not, but they will find you cold and uninviting. The moral is to switch off when finished; although it has to be admitted that this in itself is no small order. Oh to be in an institution that employs technicians to operate these machines!

If you confess your failings to the salesman when he next calls, you will end up the proud father of an automatic projector. You, in your childlike innocence, think that your problems are at an end as you carry your own little lump of heaven home. You are mistaken; they are about to be born again. Long hours of private battle lie ahead of you. You have to load each of up to fifty slides into a casette; each and everyone of which must be loaded the correct way up and in the correct order. Fifty different slides each of which can be inserted in eight different ways. Think about it qualitatively. Think about it quantitatively and come to your own decision. And if the calculations are outside your capabilities, and you are resolved to see it through, you will find yourself in a lecture theatre wanting to turn around the slide which is at present in the innermost depths of the machine. Even if the machine can be persuaded to regurgitate it, you are left with the problem of identifying which was the one you wished to turn around and how. So you decide to remove the complete cassette and think about it in the cool, away from the projector. By now you have forgotten which way you must hold a cassette to prevent the slides from falling out. When you do remember, it's the wrong way round you have remembered. Just leave all fifty slides on the floor and join in the good time now being had by all.

Our academic forefathers wrestled with epidiascopes. For the most part they didn't have to, but they did. The epidiascope is a distant cousin of the overhead projector and, in theory, utilises reflected light to project pages from books etc. In practice the light has a distinct preference for everywhere but the screen, while the heat from the arc lamp relishes its task of slowly roasting the projectionist. The projectionist's task is to keep the relevant page pressed against the machine's belly, the spring-loaded pad which once fulfilled this job having long since expired. Somehow this irrelevant page is invariably in a book which is not flat, is too big, or is laughably small; producing fuzzy, missing, or 'everything but' pictures. As we stare at the matt black and polished brass, we can easily visualise our distant ancestors shuffling their way through page after page of *Principia*; while today their heirs are busily turning roll after roll of celluloid. How times change. The machine is still befriended annually by the classics don who, giving silent assent to the age of science, happily projects a year's supply of plates of Roman pottery at an astounded audience. Alas, the epidiascope is near to extinction having been helped along the path by rapid methods of slide preparation. This is ironic as the epidiascope can, itself, be used to project slides. It is, however, rather more difficult than with a modern projector; the slides must, first of all, be correctly loaded into a slideholder which must itself be correctly loaded into the projector. Need more be said? One can't help imagining what the results must be like when a classic's don decides to employ visual aids. Totally impractical beasts, these arts people!

Instead of being simpler as one might imagine, it is frequently more difficult to make effective use of cine film than of slides. The reasons are not hard to find. A film is presented to us as a *fait accompli*, and is almost certainly not tailored to the needs of our course; with slides we can pick and choose. Film catalogues have to be hunted down and orders placed months in advance; with slides we need only wait ten seconds. We want neither the advertising content of the films from large organisations, nor their American drawl with musical backing. Excuses pure and simple. The main reason you didn't consider films was lethargy. You are a lotus-eater; nothing more. All your supposed problems have simple solutions. You don't like the commentary? Right, then, turn down the sound and give your own. If you don't like the advertising content, only show the middle portion; the bit sandwiched between the factory gardens and the chairman's chat. Be as selective as you would have been if presented with a collection of two-hundred slides. And about that film on kinetic and potential energy which has a waiting period of two years; forget about it. You should never have thought of using it. There are far more pertinent examples of the conversion of kinetic into potential energy and from potential back again to the kinetic form in every single 'Tom and Jerry' cartoon than in any straight-faced didactic production. And if Tom and Jerry are fully booked, you will find the same long-suffering beasties being twanged into and out of fences at the end of frozen lakes in many another cartoon film. If you wish, do without the 'twings' and the 'twongs' and add some of your own more weighty noises to the proceedings: there is nothing quite like a serious commentary on the trite. Explore among the other Hollywood catalogues and you will find more than enough to illustrate the *Principia* and anything you might care to say on Animal Behaviour. But keep a sense of perspective. If asked to lecture on 'The flora and fauna of the Outer Hebrides' don't drag in spinach as the excuse to show reel after reel of Popeye. Find a better excuse; spinach doesn't live in these parts. Films which have been made in university departments present fewer problems since they are short and are only too happy to get a break from long periods in the rack. This is a superficial assessment. They are indeed short, so short that no one deemed it worth while providing them with credit-titles. This can pose peculiar problems. Lecturers have been known to give the most earnest of commentaries on the movement of edge-dislocations to a film on cell differentiation. So it is best to say something that is equally applicable to dislocations, or to cells, or to anything that might obligingly fill the screen. Remarks like: 'There's another'; 'It's happening again'; and 'You saw that', are what's needed. Any dolt should be able to pass off the highly implausible as the totally credible. Those who do risk the full treatment are invariably one sequence behind that on the screen; which casts doubts on the wisdom of their having embarked on the exercise. This fault lies in spending so much time in the trees that, by the time you get around to pointing out the wood, the trees have died off – or is it vice versa? It does help to see these films through several times in advance of the lecture.

There is little point in devoting much space to the techniques of cine projection since, and this must be the cause of much heart-felt thankfulness, most of us are not let near the machines. The insurance companies say one or other of us is too great a risk. Where we are allowed we inevitably end up with a minimum of half the class around us offering ill-assorted suggestions. Suggestions such as how to form a loop of film of the required size, one which doesn't vanish when we switch on. There is the suggestion about how the lamp might be switched on simultaneously with the motor, and on how the take-up reel might be persuaded to do just that. And all the while we are martyring ourselves in yards of precious film. We soldier on. Eventually we reach the stage where the film comes off one reel, passes through the device, and successfully runs on to the other. We switch on. It appears that, commendable though this is, it does not automatically guarantee a picture. It did, however, guarantee the removal of another ten yards of sprocket holes from the film. Up to this point we have been proudly assuming the rank of, let us say, General. But now we feel that we should give younger men the opportunity to hold the reins, that they should be allowed to prove their salt. We have frankly seen enough of action and would prefer to be behind the lines. There are at least six applicants, all of whom have nursed these same machines daily from the cradle upwards. Their machines are identical to this one, even down to the letters after the model number. But there is always something fiendishly unusual about this particular one. Try boiling water on ice; it's faster. There must be no one reading this book who does not sense unbounded gratitude towards the race of projectionists who operate these machines for a living. It would therefore hardly be cricket to knock them for six; but you might just ask why the sound must always be either completely inaudible, or ear-shatteringly loud.

Although the material available at present is primarily aimed at the school market, you ought to keep one eye on the film-loop catalogues. These continuous loops, which last for several minutes, are totally contained within a plastic cassette. These cassettes must then be loaded into a special projector which is no more difficult to operate than the conventional slide projector. I can vouch for this.

All the visual aids described so far could well have kept Queen Victoria amused. But not so television. It is only recently that universities have begun spending millions on television cameras, video-recorders, projection-TV equipment; the lot. Still more recently they have begun wondering what to do with it all. Something must be done or there will be questions in the House; so committees and working parties are set up to consider and make recommendations. By far the most laudable suggestion to come out of the machinery is that the likes of you and me should video-record our winter lectures in advance. Then, when the November mists begin to thicken, we will take ourselves off to the clear air of the Bahamas; while back home among the mists our students eagerly watch us and 'The relativistic wave-mechanics of second-order pion-pion scattering'. (Of course, this will only be possible if we get paid what we are worth.) But we are skating on thin ice. Remember that other universities will be up to the same game. Somewhere there will be a veritable Fort Knox of video-tapes; the visible end products of the likes of us; us who, in all innocence, are sifting the sands with our toes as we bask in the warm Bahaman sun. All is not so idyllic back home. They have not liked us, or the way we treated the second-order pion-pion interactions. They are dissatisfied, grossly dissatisfied. They tell the Duke so. Without so much as batting an eye-lid, His Grace picks up a telephone and tells Fort Knox to send along a different tape of 'The relativistic wave-mechanics of second-order pion-pion scattering'. They do. As coolly as that our position has been usurped by Professor Wilkinson. One reel off, another on; while we, stretched out beneath our palm tree, sip another martini. The coup would not have been so bloodless had we been there in person. Perhaps we should have stayed at home instead. Then we could have donned appropriate disguise and mingled with the students after the lecture, proclaiming 'Damn good lectures these'. That would have stopped the discontent.

Not much need be said about the techniques of being video-recorded since at least a half-dozen producers, floor managers, and make-up girls will have come along as part of the package deal. They will have much to say. The big new challenge for us is how to effectively use a close-up of a twitching nose or a fluttering eyebrow.

We are not yet through with visual aids.

CHAPTER

8

Demonstrations

Demonstrations originate in preparation rooms. Preparation rooms adjoin the larger lecture theatres of the older universities. Enter such a preparation room and you are met by glass-fronted cases, each almost three feet deep and each stretching to near ceiling level. On top of the cases live Fletcher and the wave-model. All the rest is kept under lock and some key or other.

On one shelf you spot the electrophorus which someone rubbed every year to impress a mystified class. He has retired now and the electrophorus is unlikely to be rubbed again. On this shelf are also a collection of evacuated glass tubes each perching proudly on its turned mahogany pedestal. The tubes contain Maltese Crosses and rotating vanes, and still have the capacity to amuse audiences. Then there is the X-ray tube which saw service in a field hospital during the First World War and which, if the brass plate be believed, was presented to the university by someone whose name now means nothing. The apparatus of an even earlier generation is stored on the shelf above. At odd moments various people come in and try to guess the purpose of it all. Was that contraption with coils and compass-needle for determining a ship's magnetic axis? Or is it an obsolete type of galvanometer? And what could those perforated discs have been for? One guess is as good as another. There is less uncertainty about the adjacent 'Heat and Mechanics' cupboard where Bunsen, Atwood and Kater can be clearly distinguished. Those are obviously a collection of telescopes

and that's a cardboard box full of Helmholtz resonators in
'Optics and Sound'. Also to be found here are the dissectable
plaster models of the ear and eye in their fading reds and
blues. The plaster is cracking, but several Latin names still
half-adhere.

Many of us at the newer universities evoke some such
picture as our private excuse for not having lecture demonstrations. When pressed further we protest that our course
is so swinging that lecture demonstrations are 'out'. We are
all photoelectric effect (a particularly unfortunate example)
and interatomic forces (not much better). We teach special
relativity instead of Kater (still getting nowhere) and general
relativity instead of Boyle (keep trying). Even if you can find
only four topics a term to demonstrate on, so much the
better: the fewer there are, the greater will be their impact!
So lecture demonstrations are 'in', although you may be
absolutely right to avoid the more musty examples.

Superficially, the simplest type of demonstration to mount
is the one which merely aims to show specimens to the
audience. No matter how imaginative the course, the biologist or geologist will still have to flourish the odd example.
The geologist may itch to show off his rock collection and
the engineer may long to exhibit the innards of his valves.
Both have to learn that their specimens are mute and must
be made to speak for themselves.

The first, and most common, failing of some lecturers is
to leave all their specimens on the bench throughout the
lecture. What happens is that mention of the word 'granite'
or 'triode' causes them to make some involuntary gesture in
the general direction of several dozens of something. They
then continue as if nothing had happened; until the words
'flint' or 'pentode' occur, when they are seized with fresh
convulsions. Later it's 'sandstone' and 'heptode' that bring
on the attacks. To begin with the audience finds it vaguely
titillating to know that somewhere among the collection is
the relevant rock or valve. So they give a cursory glance in
the direction of the convulsions; in much the same way that

half the populace will look up at the sky if one does. The novelty soon wears off.

The slightly more determined don will make a hectic rush at the pile, dive feverishly into it, and emerge clutching something which he solemnly declares to be the said granite or triode. For all the audience know, he could indeed be telling the truth. Such lecturers are at least starting to hold the right end of the stick, but the effect would have been greater had they kept their specimens out of view until required. The audience would then be kept wondering if there are any more to come; and it's always an achievement to keep an audience in suspense. It's the technique of the television housewife who must dive into her washing machine to produce the linen which has been stewing in something novel. Keep it hidden till required, and then declare what can be seen. But don't keep them posted about what can't be seen! You are still a long way from letting the audience sense the stone's texture or examine the tube's innards.

Most lecturers now think they have the cat in the bag. They will pass the specimen around to allow the audience to 'have a look at it'. If only they did. No sooner has it got beyond the first row than they embark on something new. By the time it has reached the back row the subject of the lecture is stellar structure or television camera-work. Those aware of this hazard try to circumvent it by first preaching to the class for a good ten minutes on what to expect when the specimen does reach them. Then the specimen is released and the lecturer holds his peace. And sure enough, when it does reach them they have forgotten wthether they are supposed to be looking at a stone or a valve. They turn it over a few times and, shaking their heads, toss it on. To counter this unexpected new hazard, the lecturer decides to simultaneously launch ten copies of the sample on its travels. But each person is now so frustrated at having to look at the same thing ten times over that they fail to notice that the eleventh, the twenty-first and the thirty-first are different from the first. Their frustration, however, is nothing compared to that of the fellow at the far end of the back row who finds himself slowly disappearing behind a mountain of stones, or being built into some novel electronic device. The whole performance can all too easily develop into a sort of children's party game. All we need now is a piano.

What you really need is a television camera capable of taking close-ups and some large-screen sets. Not only will this allow the audience to see the fine detail, but, much more important, it can fuse you, the specimen, and the audience together. This fusion will occur if, and only if, the audience become as engrossed in the specimen as do you. So turn the specimen round and round, get clues, pick out features like intrusions, have second thoughts and then muse on the significance of it all. Any audience will readily hook on to someone who is 'discovering' things in front of their eyes. Needless to say the tactic should be varied; another time the principal features might be pointed out with a pencil while you employ a staccato commentary to match. In either variant avoid rushing headlong into detail. If the audience are never shown the complete object on the screen they will view it directly and persistently, although the temptation to watch 'live' may be reduced by having the sets close by you. You, of course, will have to keep one eye on a screen and one on the specimen. A not unimportant point is that many television sets omit a high frequency whistle which you may not notice, but which can dement the class. To eliminate this whistle, you often have to switch the set off: turning down the brightness is inadequate. Blank raster lines can also prove very distracting.

Should television not be available, an overhead projector can be used quite effectively to blow-up either translucent objects or pieces that can profitably be studied in silhouette; e.g. the electrode arrangement of many valves show up well when placed on the glass plate of such projectors, and if the valves can be 'broken' apart, so much the better. A transparent ruler will indicate the scale of things. The shapes of objects such as crystals and the texture of surfaces may often be made clearer by exploiting the fact that light is reflected and scattered when a specimen is placed in a strong light beam: you simply hold it several inches in front of the lens of an unloaded slide projector. But whatever your sleight of hand, the specimen must come to life: if it fails to do so, the audience might just as well, and more readily, have been shown a few slides.

Geographers, chemists and medical people will frequently resort to talking about wall-charts. Again, the advice is the same as when dealing with slides, or on any other static projected image, such as from projection microscopes. Don't put it up before it is required and take it down once you have finished. Do spend a few seconds on the general features before jumping on the fleas; if the audience are denied this information they will never develop an itch for your details. Make the resolution to ignore minutiae of no pressing interest to the class. And remember that the class, unless they have duplicates in front of them, may wish to copy down what is on the canvas. Either allow time for them to do so or, and perhaps this is often preferable, put up a simplified sketch on the board. Similar remarks apply, of course, to presenting 'live' specimens. Many a nervous beginner shows off his pet to the class for five seconds, says he is sure they have 'got it down', and is then mystified by all the mirth. And it's not only beginners who make this boob. With more experience you may merely dismiss the laughter with greater equanimity.

You might think that dynamic demonstrations employing standard commercial equipment should present few problems. Yet many lecturers are quite capable of launching straight into something (the experiment presumably) without indicating the vital components, or saying which dials read what. The audience hear the words 'I'll show you' but all they behold is a twittering meter and some mute pulling rheostats. Then follows 'well it worked' and the experience is over. Some one person is satisfied. It's probably the old story of all his personality being sunk lock, stock and barrel in that rheostat; he has nothing left over. It is indeed difficult to give a grossly over-simplified description with your tongue of what is a much more complex piece of equipment at your fingertips. It takes courage to be able to say of an oscilloscope that it 'simply measures voltages', or whatever, while you are struggling with the trigger-level knob and a dozen others. The temptation is to tell them all or nothing. Because of this, spend some time planning out in advance the exact words to be spoken, and when; and what vital parts will be pointed out; and how. Those meters; will they be large enough to be seen from the back row? And if they are, how can they then be seen by people at the sides of the class? So I will remember to twist the meters back and forth (if I have none of the projection type). Then if a vital component, e.g. a photoelectric cell, is buried deep in the apparatus, shouldn't I have a second one to show the class? And how? Would it not be better still to have just the one and to assemble the circuit from scratch? And if minor technical reasons make the actual circuit more complex than the one on the board, will I bluff them? Anyway, how can they see what I am doing? So is there any point in assembling it? Will I tell them what to expect or will I let it come as a surprise? Should I interchange the conventional order of prediction followed by the proving experiment? Should I not occasionally 'do' experiments which don't work, and then examine why? How about experiments which shouldn't work but do? Will I keep the apparatus hidden until required, or will the change as it becomes dynamic be adequate? What will I say during the agonising minute while the Polaroid projection film is developing?

These and a great many other questions should occur to you. Think about them before you walk in. If you simply trust that all will be well on the day, it won't. It never is. And if these are not your sort of questions, then you may learn something from watching good television presenters.

Notice how they omit the finer details (at least to begin with); how they make very definitive points with a pencil or finger as they speak; and guess how many times they must have rehearsed the experiment before the broadcast began.

In my opinion, some of the most successful demonstrations are those which employ highly unorthodox and often cheap pieces of equipment. Quite apart from the cost factor, a strong case may be made against employing off-the-shelf commercial apparatus. The students know that it must work, otherwise the manufacturer would be out of business: if the apparatus doesn't work it is solely due to our incompetence. Besides the superficial sameness of much of this equipment must, impact-wise, lead to ever diminishing returns. It has none of the glamour of real life laboratories. It's all too prim and proper. Let's have an example of the dangers of orthodoxy.

In the dull, uncompromising world of 'Properties of Matter' courses, there are but four solid materials. All physics students know them to be copper, brass, iron and lead. To judge by the demonstrations, copper alone conducts heat; brass alone extends under stress; iron alone expands on heating; and only lead will swing at the end of a simple pendulum. Our lecturer tells his class that he now wants to 'move on to do' Newton's Law of Universal Gravitation. What happens? Just watch him. He declares with a rare degree of enthusiasm that 'this is the apparatus' and the audience, who have been gazing at it for the past three-quarters of an hour, are vaguely shown the very two spheres of lead (yes, it's our old friend lead) which have been at the centre of their thoughts for some considerable time. Now, the lead spheres hang on the end of something. They are told its name but that is all. They are shown two more lead spheres which, likewise, had not escaped their attention. The experiment is 'done' without much further ado. Not surprisingly it worked since it has that seal of guarantee; the metal name-plate of an old established firm. And throughout not a word of mention was made of why spheres, why lead, and even why this particular balance was employed. Such questions as these occurred to neither lecturer nor students. It was all a *fait accompli*. No preliminary experimentation was undertaken to justify this extremely sophisticated set-up.

Try this for a change. You hold, say, a turnip in one hand and give a member of the audience any other object which comes to hand, e.g. a bag of coal, a lettuce, or a white rabbit. Ask him to bring his object up towards your turnip. Does he feel any pull? Do I? Bring it up closer. Any pull? No? So what? We shall try and make things more sensitive then. Let's hang the turnip on a chemical balance and bring the bag of coal underneath it. Still no effect. So what? This (mock-up) torsion balance is more sensitive still. ('I know, because if I blow . . .'). Let's try again. But perhaps we might see something if we used more massive objects and brought them closer together. This would suggest spheres or cylinders of high density material. And so on. The gain in appreciation of scientific methodology is enormous and we have achieved it with only supermarket materials. The audience are kept guessing whether the next stage of refinement will show any effect.

The critic will be quick to point out that if these techniques are employed wholesale very little material can be 'got through'. No it is not being suggested that prior to performing every experiment you should trace its design history. What is being suggested is that, at least occasionally, you should get out of the rut of conventional demonstration experiments. Perhaps a design study is appropriate to the major classical experiments: perhaps you should be unorthodox when conventional demonstrations are ill-understood, or when you wish to demonstrate your faith. There are many sides to our faith which we should demonstrate more often, e.g. if you really believe that gravitational attraction is not just transient, drop several dozen bricks at irregular intervals in the course of the lecture. If you really believe that a chemical reaction is translation-independent perform it twice, once at the front of the theatre and once at the back. If you believe it is mass independent, do it in the microgram and the bath tub ranges. If you really believe in the 'conversion' of mechanical energy to heat energy, don't only demonstrate it using the one standard apparatus with its brass drum and its canvas brake. Instead get a heavy packing case and push it back and forth across the theatre floor. Get down and crawl around the floor, feel it, and report on your findings. Now try and fry an egg on it. This is testing your faith, and it only takes a couple of minutes. If you can find no convincing argument why $'weight = mg'$, climb up a step-ladder with a vase of flowers hanging from the end of your tie. No one will ever forget the argument; and that should please your critics. Above all, bubble over. The audience will start simmering also, but they can only come to the boil if the experiments are at their level of appreciation: which may be yet another argument for the unorthodox. Many conventional experiments are either conceptually too difficult, or have too much associated paraphernalia. A swaying pendulum is the last way any normal person would dream of measuring the acceleration of a free falling object! Nor do you need a radar station to discover that birds migrate.

Not the least argument for the unorthodox is that the materials are cheap and expendable. Supermarket goods are, however, definitely best kept out of view until required. If, for example, you have a celluloid duck on the bench the audience will know you are going to take a bath (but please not to demonstrate Archimedes); they will also keep a book on just when!

Many subjects allow topics to be usefully demonstrated by means of simulators. A classic example is in the electron-optics where the behaviour of an electron in an electric field may be simulated by a ball-bearing running up and down appropriate hills and valleys. Here the danger is not that you will have no luck at playing with ball-bearings, but rather that you will fail to discuss the link between the simulator and the simulated. Unless the nature of the analogue is discussed, the weaker student will, in this particular example, think that inside valves are hills and valleys which electrons run up and down! They find it difficult to convert the visual gravitational potential energy into unseen electrical potential energy – possibly because most of them have no idea what is meant by potential energy. Unless you are aware of every possible misinterpretation and are prepared to bear these in mind when planning your commentary, it may be best to steer clear of these simulators.

Naturally, there is plenty of room for unorthodox simulators. If the laboratory does not possess, or cannot afford, the usual vibrator-driven gas simulator, buy a couple of dozen balls from Woolworths, put them in a shallow box, and vibrate it rapidly up and down above your head. If the laboratory cannot afford even this, wave your fists about in the air and go berserk around the theatre. And if you want to simulate diffusion in a liquid have two lots of ten to twenty volunteers down the front and allow them to jostle together. The physical-chemistry of diffusion will soon be apparent. This is a far superior simulator to one employing ball-bearings. The repulsive force between two humans in contact more closely approximates that between two atoms than does the sharp repulsive force between hard bearings. With enough volunteers you can simulate all of chemical kinetics. The human body is a good 'atom', and a cheap one!

Apart from lecture theatre demonstrations, most of us will be expected to 'demonstrate' in practical classes although, in our formative years, we will not be entrusted with the responsibility of setting up the class experiments. It might not be tactful to enquire who did conceive the first-year class which we have been asked to take charge of. Whoever it was, it all happened a long time ago. Strange how it is that so many of the first-year classes in our universities have such a family-likeness. Perhaps he, whoever he was, was a nomad who wandered from campus to campus offering advice for a moderate fee. Perhaps he ran a firm of consultants. Perhaps he wrote a book, or manual, 'on Practical Class Experiments'. Perhaps he managed a company which manufactured convenient apparatus.

The great art in running practical classes is to busy yourself away in one corner beneath a pile of books which urgently need marking. Any queries directed at you are quickly referred to postgraduate demonstrators who are there to assist: after a couple of classes such queries should have dried up. You, of course, must never set about discovering how much the postgraduates themselves know. You can only hope that the experiments are each accompanied by detailed instructions fastened between sheets of glass; the kind of instructions which, in the manner of medieval prints, identifies all the components as $a, b, c, \ldots$ and which gives precise instructions on which lever to pull, and how, and on which meter to read and when, instructions which show what headed columns to draw and which tell the reader exactly how to proceed with the totals of these columns; instructions which show him what graph to draw and tell him what the gradient represents; instructions which may be within the grasp of the postgraduates themselves, and which they will read aloud to the enquirer as, together, they grope around. Just the techniques to convert our chicks into battery hens.

You have enough on your own plate. You have a written-up experiment before you, but take heart. Don't attempt to understand the experiment. Look at the last line and see if he has put in any errors. Errors are the great thing. If he has none, don't consider the script any further. If he has some, see if he has quoted his result to more significant figures than is justified. Should he have an excess of figures, write him a long essay calculated to undermine his confidence in humanity. Should he have the right number of figures, have another look at his error. Maybe he has stated his error as $\pm.063$. Ah! Now you can go to town and ask him, in a foot-note, if he is certain of the last '3'. Should he have been naughty enough to approximate his error to $\pm\cdot05$, pose the query of what is the error of his error. Keep on pressing ever deeper; you always win out in the end. Firmly fix your eyes on the last line and all else will pale to insignificance. Errors are the thing: or yields; or their signatures; or the date and bench number; or the width of the margin; or the type of paper. You name it; the choice is yours.

The proper running of a practical class demands that you first perform all the experiments yourself and then insist on each postgraduate performing at least a couple of them. As in straight lecturing, there are no short-cuts to success. This is particularly so in practical work where we have to get to grips with the eccentricities of the laboratory's particular burettes, resistance-boxes or power-supplies. You can only advise on, and discuss, what you yourself have attempted! Then it is simply man-to-man chatting.

CHAPTER
9
Tutorials

There is a diffuse rumbling on the door but we dismiss it as the wind and continue cleaning our nails. The desk behind which we are seated is opposite the door; a substantial desk with a top of veneered plywood and a modesty panel. The rumbling persists. We drop the nail file on to the desk and reach a hand around to close the window. It is firmly shut. How strange. Our thoughts return to the door. It dawns.

'Come in.'

From where we are seated we can see that the door handle is turning cautiously. We understand what this means. Four very sheepish individuals enter and the front two legs of our chair land smartly on the lino-covered floor.

'And what can we do for you?'

In retrospect it will become clear that this was a singularly foolish question to put, particularly to these four. But the damage has been done.

'We have come for our tutorial,' declares their leader. A good ten seconds pass before we feel the impact of this suggestion. We press our feet against the modesty panel and the desk moves forward. We stand up, stretch ourselves, and make for the radiator. Something is bothering us. It's the implicit hint that they are expecting a tutorial which upsets us. Tutorials? We cast our mind forward and backwards, and then a bit sideways, but without much immediate success. Then, quite out of the blue, we recall having heard someone in the tea-room mention something about tutorials. Yes, we remember reading somewhere in one of the university handbooks, we forget which one, that the university has a tutorial system! That, unlike other universities, here it is the kernel of the university's teaching methods. That 'it provides an intellectually stimulating relationship between tutor and student and gives the student a firm sense of "oneness" with intellectual thought within the university'. Now we realise why four very sheepish individuals are standing just inside the open door.

'Ah yes, you have come for your tutorial on the relativistic wave-mechanics of second-order pion-pion interactions,' we affirm, demonstrating the powers of intellectual thought within this university. They exchange shaggy looks with each other, and all speak at once.

'Oh no. It's on non-equilibrium statistical thermodynamics.'

The suggestion is so preposterous that we choose to disregard it. We take our right leg off the radiator, lean our head back till it touches the notice-board, and smile broadly.

'Oh no. There must be some mistake.'

The smile bursts forth as we realise that victory is ours. We take several deliberate paces to the desk, retrieve the nail file, and slip it into our pocket where we thumb its surface. But more sheepish looks are exchanged. One, whom we suspect is female, reaches into the pocket of a coat which possibly belonged to its grandmother in the 1920s and produces an irregularly folded piece of paper. It is unfolded with considerable difficulty and handed over. We examine it, but choose to ignore the knowing glances which each sheep passes to the other. The thing lifts a palsied arm and indicates some small square on the heavily-creased sheet. We recollect what day of the week it is and confirm the time on our watch. Then we check that the time-table is for this term. It is. We are compelled to murmur that the name printed in that square does correspond with what we remember ours as, and that the subject of the tutorial is non-equilibrium statistical thermodynamics.

'It must be the computer. The programme is riddled with errors. It has put in the wrong Walton.'

We expand at length on this theme. The time-tables are now entrusted to computers, but computers must be programmed, and the programmers, being human, are fallible. These programmers are therefore not above making mistakes. They have been known to make mistakes; they do so frequently. In fact they are a right collection of morons. To our very great pleasure the four warm to this assessment of the situation. They enjoy learning of the weaknesses of the flesh. They are on our side.

We slide around and slip off the desk and make for the telephone. Let it be confessed, we are simply presuming that there is another Walton tucked away somewhere. There must be; ours is a modern university with many hundreds of faculty members and more so of administrators. We thumb about near the end of the directory. It luckily confirms our hunch. There is one with initials D.R.M. As fast as our index finger will move, we ring up D.R.M. and inform him that, owing to the damn incompetence of the programmers, we have his tutorial group right here in the room with us. We ask if we should send them over right away or, if he would care to suggest an alternative time, we will gladly pass this on to the four.

In the course of our conversation with D.R.M. we learn that his major preoccupation in life is the pigmentation of Indonesian barks. It is with some reluctance that we assent to his view that non-equilibrium statistical thermodynamics is a closer relative of pions than of Indonesian barks. With even greater reluctance we take a more charitable view of computer programmers than hitherto. As we click the phone back on its receiver we sense that the four have overheard D. R. M. Walton's personal opinion of us.

We invite the four to pull up chairs and make themselves at home. We suggest a semi-circle as an appropriate arrangement. If they wish to, they can hang their coats on the peg behind the door. One accepts the offer. We pick up a duster and proceed to clean the board. We clean it ever so slowly, ever so methodically, yet somehow fail to notice that it has already been washed free from every trace of chalk by the cleaners the previous evening. As we cover the board in a thin veil of whiteness, we search for a reason why the dice should be loaded so heavily against us. Then before our eyes we can dimly see that P.S. which the professor added to his letter of last October. Something about there being a possibility that we might be asked to give a couple of hours' tutorials in addition to the lecture course. The possibility has become an actuality.

We deem this to be an appropriate occasion for extended introductions laying particular stress on the importance of really getting to know each other. Intellectual integrity, after all, demands 'oneness'. So we commence a detailed analysis of each and everyone's educational backgrounds. What primary schools did we attend? What were the science teachers like? Anyone against comprehensive education? How came we to go to university? But the four are not to be drawn and only five minutes of our sixty have passed. There is a deep hush as they stare vacantly at the scored lino squares, scored, no doubt, when an earlier tutor in- vited his four to pull up their chairs. What a shame we served up the history of the university as an *hors d'oeuvre* to our first lecture. That would have provided their susten- ance now.

Then, quite unheralded and without any encouragement from us, the chap sitting on the right of the thing from the 1920s reaches into the pocket of his PVC jacket and pro- duces a folded exercise book. He unfolds it and we read the legend 'Lancashire Education Authority. Newtontown Grammar School. French Prose.' He thumbs the over- thumbed corners and opening it up where the French prose ends, thrusts it into our unwilling hands, demanding we tell him where that came from. The 'that' in question reads:

$$\Sigma \mu_i \varepsilon_i (1 - \beta)/kT = \mathcal{N}.$$

Need we say more?

Oxbridge dons know how to escape from such situations, but reasons of high principle, or low finance, preclude us from keeping a bottle of sherry and four or five glasses at the ready to counter these assaults. At our university this privilege belongs to the Duke and the professors who both employ it freely and to good effect.

When in a tight corner invoke principles. We do. The high principle that they are wasting their time attempting to understand why

$$\Sigma\mu_i\varepsilon_i(1 - \beta)/kT=\mathcal{N}$$

if they have no idea why the sky is blue, or why the grass is green. Or anything that we are qualified to *ad lib* on. We *ad lib* away, trusting they find us as intellectually stimulating as we find ourselves. There is a good chance that they won't know why the sky is blue or why the grass is green, and there is the complete certainty that in their eyes we epitomise the pinnacle of intellectual thought within this university. But, and let's be honest, there are bounds to our intellectual thoughts. We must therefore steer the four away from the blue sky to the safer domain of second-order pion-pion interactions. The transition is easily accomplished for we have by now soared to realms above theirs. In the unlikely event that one is still airborne we merely remind him (although it is scarcely necessary) that pions inhabit the furthermost depths of the blue. So we proudly march to the filing cabinet offering, as we go, our profuse thanks to the owner of the Newtontown Grammar School exercise book for raising such a thought-provoking question: a question we shall return to when we have covered the necessary ground work. We pull out our lecture notes on 'The relativistic wave-mechanics of second-order pion-pion interactions', slam the drawer shut, and return to our armchair. We have adequate material for the rest of the term's tutorials on non-equilibrium statistical thermodynamics.

Just suppose we had no lecture course to our credit. We must forge ahead, but how? Why, we would tell them of our research work. They would be left in no doubt that our work on β-brass or the energy levels of iridium are a particularly fine example of

$$\Sigma\mu_i\varepsilon_i(1-\beta)/kT=\mathcal{N}.$$

The connection between the two, and hence the problem which arose after the French Prose, will become abundantly clear as we examine the mysteries of β-brass. And examine them we do. We examine the problems of building a He^3 cryostat; the problems of heat conduction; the problems of leaks. The leak detector is a recent acquisition. It cost £20,000 and is in continual use. Before the days of this machine we had to use a Tesla Coil and paint the glassware with alcohol. It was very unreliable, insensitive and seldom sorted out the problem at hand.

Under normal conditions either one of these techniques is more than adequate to meet all contingencies. However, I have had occasion to cope with high-minded individuals who maintained that they had a divine right to know why

$$\Sigma\mu_i\varepsilon_i(1-\beta)/kT=\mathcal{N}.$$

This in itself was not alarming. What was alarming was their insistence that they should be told why. It was only after they threatened an interview with the professor that I began to take their claims seriously. 'Of course you have every right to know why

$$\Sigma\mu_i\varepsilon_i(1-\beta)/kT=\mathcal{N},$$

and a lot more besides,' said I.

My question about who was giving this lecture course unfortunately only brought the professor's name back to the fore. A pity, because the usual tactic of damning the lecturer responsible for such an over-sophisticated course would have backfired had these high-minded individuals persisted with their threat. It would likewise have been sailing too near the wind to suggest that the 'non-equilibrium statistical' part of the course's title crept in by error. Under the circumstances there was nothing for it but to say all that was known on the subject of 'non-equilibrium statistical thermodynamics'. This was the problem. But for a stroke of good fortune which brought to mind the techniques of the Church, it would have remained unsolved. I saw before me, not the title of a lecture course, but a text on which many a good sermon could, and most certainly would, be preached. These sermons would offer detailed textual criticism.

With our elbows resting on the broad teak arms of the chair we attempt to bounce the outstretched fingers of our right hand off the outstretched fingers of our left hand. We partially succeed and remark that any understanding of non-equilibrium must stem from an appreciation of equilibrium. As we shall shortly demonstrate, the very word 'equilibrium' carries with it a wealth of symbolism. We commence our quest by removing a book from the shelf beside the filing cabinet. We lay it flat on the floor in front of our feet. We lift up one corner of the book and let go. It slaps the floor. We lift up the next corner and let go. Then the third corner and finally the fourth. The effect is the same. To lend force to our suggestions we repeat the operation tilting it about each side in turn. Then we put it to the four that they may have noticed something.

'That's called stable equilibrium.'

We deem this to be important enough to warrant a trip to the board to write up 'stable equilibrium'. We suggest they copy it down. We look at our watches. We tell them of the common error of spelling stable 'stabile' and how when, as a sixth-former, we wrote that a chemical we had analysed in semi-micro analysis was 'stabile' the master wrote 'spelling not very stable'.

We return not to our armchair but to the desk, and to its top right-hand drawer. After rummaging about beneath the envelopes and circulars, during which we spot that our aspirin bottle is empty, we emerge with one of last season's tennis balls. Resisting the temptation to quote the bit of Shakespeare we once knew, we roll the ball around on the floor. Four pairs of eyes follow its sparse green hair and 'Neutral Equilibrium' is soon within their grasp. So too is the fact that we once tutored Virginia Wade, who is staging a comeback.

'Anyone like me to go over neutral equilibrium again?'

Regrettably all are quite happy and none have any problems.

Which brings us to the nub of the course: non-equilibrium. The pencil we are looking for takes some finding and fortunately it has a broken point. We re-sharpen it as lovingly as any craftsman could. We sense its fine tip and stand it upright on the veneered hardboard, catching it before it quite reaches the horizontal. The experiment is repeated again, and again, and yet again. The *ne plus ultra* of 'non-equilibrium' has been approached. So ends our first tutorial. For their next tutorial they must think up four examples of each types of equilibrium.

For our next tutorial we made sure that we arrived a goodly ten minutes late and remembered to mutter something about Sir George being slow to leave. Then followed the twenty-two-minute recap of the salient points met in the last tutorial. After this we invited each goat to disclose its own four examples of the three types of equilibrium. As they unburdened their souls we listened most intently; where was that ill-chosen example which would prove they had understood nothing of what we said last week, which would justify a retreat from the world? But they had grasped it. Now we understand why Jonah was exceedingly displeased with the people of Nineveh.

'Statistics' presents us with untold possibilities; we can see our way through the remaining twenty minutes of this second tutorial. We play darts against the blackboard with pieces of chalk. We toss coins. We ask them what is the probability that two of them have grandmothers of the same age; they can think about this rather tricky one for next time when, unless we hear to the contrary, we will assume they have found the answer. We point out the statistical link between smoking and cancer; between air-polution and bronchitis, and the four grow convinced that there is something to 'statistics' after all. The qualitative spirit of our approach has been appreciated.

Which leaves us with 'thermodynamics' to fill out the last six tutorials of the term. Let's count our blessings; long ago we attended a course of six lectures on 'The Steam Engine' and, if our memory is not at fault, these machines are pure thermodynamics. Enthalpy, entropy, Helmholtz free energy are all to be found between the fire-box and the track. Should these qualities not raise their enthusiasm we have page after page of Steam Tables that must surely do the trick. And, because they don't own Steam Tables, we regretfully cannot set any written work. So wide has the road opened up that we should never get side-tracked into discussing the sheet of problems that their lecturer has been inconsiderate enough to distribute. Reader, never let it be said that you cannot cope with tutorials!

I will however conclude this chapter on a slightly more serious note. Unlike lectures, which are primarily subject-centred and which are unlikely to alter in character if the attendance changes from one hundred to five hundred, tutorials must be student-centred and will certainly alter if the numbers change from one to five. To lecture successfully you must understand Everyman; to tutor successfully you must also understand the extremes of humanity. Not being intimate with your particular one or five, it would be highly presumptious to suggest what form 'your' tutorials should take. Mini-lectures, or even shoulder-weeping sessions, may be what is required. Human understanding and a certain sleight-of-hand are the prerequisites.

If I may be permitted one specific recommendation, it is Be Prepared. If the tutorial is timed to complement a particular lecture course, attend it; but only if the lecturer is convinced that he can completely ignore your presence. Try telling him how much you appreciate half-truths, how you relish unsophisticated arguments, and what a joy it is to be able to go somewhere incognito. But if he persists in playing up to you, then go away and get to work on his course outline; an exercise which will involve you in the same sort of spade-work as would planning a lecture course. Perhaps because the preliminaries are so similar you may now feel like serving up your erudition in lecture style. It may be the only way you know of spreading the muck, but in nine cases out of ten it will be the wrong way. As soon as that lad in PVC asks you why

$$\Sigma \mu_i \varepsilon_i (1 - \beta)/kT = N,$$

don't give him the answer on a plate. Make him sing for his supper; first solo and then as a duet. Get someone else to accompany him while you dangle carrots before both their eyes. Suggest they have the relation upside-out and inside-down and, once they agree with you, remember it should be downside-up and outside-in. Careful though; it could all be a cunning trap. Never mind, two can play at this game. . . .

'Anyone know why the sky is green?'

CHAPTER

10

Seminars, colloquia, symposia and such-like

These are a highly specialised race of things. You can, however, in complete safety ignore anything that the *Oxford Dictionary* may have to say about one being different from t'other. 'Taint true. They are all the same; a speaker (you) and an audience (a dozen).

But how came you to be here? There are several possibilities. Firstly, that 'here' maybe your old university (X, say). There (at X, say) one professor, busily stirring a crockery cupful of laboratory tea, was foolish enough to remark to another professor:

'Remember that young chap Walton? Whatever did he spend his three years doing?'

As he spoke, he flexed the plastic spoon against the bottom of his cup, crushing what remained of the sugar into nothingness. Whereupon the second professor, who was experiencing some difficulty with removing the wrapper from his wafer biscuit while keeping hold of the cup with his other hand, chuckled back:

'No idea. Better have him down to give a seminar.'

That's one possibility, but not the only one. The reason you are now at university Y could simply be that they got hold of X's list of seminars, with the express intention of compiling their own list. The young dogs-body with the honorary job of arranging colloquia has spotted your name.

'See this? Some chap has been speaking on "The Fermi

Surface of the α-form of β-brass". That's another Monday filled.'

He has heard the words 'Fermi Surface' being flung around his department, so he may be forgiven for imagining the subject to be of some interest to the members of Y. The rub is that this process is highly contagious; which could explain why you are now at Z.

Let's not be cynical. The real reason that you are now at X, Y or Z is that the abstract of your paper in *The Proceedings of the Littlepool Physical Society (Section A) 78, 137-139* has been noted.

If you have had your wits about you, you will have arrived in time for lunch. There the relevant professor will have mustered, with the bribe of a free meal (sherry included), the half-dozen or so who claimed even the remotest interest in either brasses or Fermi Surfaces. Some of these claimants will have come as a distinct surprise to the professor. You, of course, will be duly impressed by the size of the following, but will be prudent enough to avoid even mentioning β-brasses or Fermi Surfaces. They will ask you if so-and-so is doing any useful work these days (he isn't), and whether U.G.C. has frozen Stage IV of the department's extensions (they have). You will ask them if they have had student riots also (they have), and whether S.R.C. has coughed up the money for their accelerator (they haven't). And at some stage between the sherry and the port you will carefully plant that plum anecdote about how a comment of yours started Shoenberg off on Fermi Surfaces: the plum which the professor will swallow and then cough up in his opening remarks introducing you at the seminar. A sure way of establishing your reputation among the upstart research students who haven't got around to reading your papers yet.

In his opening remarks, the professor will also mention that it is a very real pleasure to welcome you (back) and how much he, who is surely speaking on behalf of all, appreciates your being able to fit in this talk. If there are a

few snow flakes about, you will be painted as a latter-day
Hannibal, and if you contrive to sprain your ankle the
audience will learn that you have come along against the
wishes of Harley Street. A few hands will clap and you will
quit the front row where you have been seated in solitary
splendour, walk to the bench and return the pleasures. It
is much too delicate to advise on whether to field a return
anecdote. You alone must make this decision, on the basis
of whether or not the professor may have heard of Stephen
Potter, Esq. Don't forget the privilege of burying Caesar
will be his. But right now it's your privilege.

This is the moment to rapidly assess your audience. The
professor we have already mentioned. By now he will have
returned to the front row where, attempting to keep his head
vertical, he proceeds to draft long-overdue letters, and perhaps to turn over in his mind the question calculated to
devastate you at the end of the talk; although, as has been
said, much depends on his acquaintance with Stephen Potter. At ill-chosen intervals he will stare half-wittingly at
you and your scribbles, nod, and return to more pressing
matters. Then who else is there? There are the six you met
at lunch and who are feeling under some sort of obligation
to attend. Better watch these; they are the type who slip out
the rear door when your back is turned. Glare at them, the
door, and at them again: let them know you have read their
souls. Then there are the professor's research students who
are there to be seen by him. But they don't count for they
couldn't tell an α-brass from an ω-one. Also here to be seen
by the professor is the would-be-up-and-coming young lecturer who later hopes to demonstrate his dexterity when it
is time for discussion. He will be your biggest headache.
Seated up at the back of the theatre is an elderly gentleman
who once lectured the professor as an undergraduate but,
being a gentleman, missed out in the promotion stakes. He
is here to foster the illusion that he still leads the vanguard
of research. Fear not; experience should have taught him
never to ask questions, but should he put any, the professor,

not you, will quickly *reductio ad absurdem* them. All you
need do is display whose side you are on. This clearly depends on whether or not you are chasing the senior lectureship which the professor's department is currently advertising. Now let's be generous. There will also be the one or
two who have a genuine desire to find out all they can about
the Fermi Surface of the α-form of β-brass. They are easily
distinguished for they carry large cloth-covered ring-folders
packed to overflowing. The rings will snap and re-snap every
so often. Very reassuring. It is the thirst of these one or two
you will try and satisfy. No, which you will succeed in
quenching.

For the benefit of the lay-reader, it is perhaps well to explain that the subject of the seminar lies in the depths of
solid-state physics. It is concerned with the subtler aspects
of electrical conduction in alloys. That being so, you would
think it safe to assume that all present will have heard of
alloys and be aware of what conduction is. Well, wouldn't
you? Not so with 99.9 per cent of seminar-givers. Indeed
the ninety and nine (and point nine) per cent will, for the
first five minutes, treat the audience as congenital idiots
who have never heard of brass, let alone electrons. They will
tell them how the ancient Romans discovered brass, and
show slides of Julius Caesar. They will reveal that an ancient
Greek once rubbed a cat with amber, and their names and
dates will be written bold and clear on the board. They
will lay bare their own experiences with cats and tell of
their holidays in Athens. Then, without any warning whatever, without so much as an inkling, they will launch straight
into the innermost innards of Fermi Surfaces. Without so
much as an excuse-me or the vaguest of hints as to what a
Fermi Surface might happen to be. The likes of us are left
wondering whether it's a term in symbolic logic or a part
of our anatomy. And the likes of them won't surface at
all in the next fifty-five minutes.

You who have been taking the message of this book to
heart will make no such mistakes. True, you may spend the

first half-hour setting the scene so that what you intend saying in the last half-hour will be understandable to everyone in this broad field. Yes, to all. Not just to the person who shares your bench or laboratory. Perhaps you should aim at the second-year research student. It all depends on local conditions, so these are worth finding out. Naturally you will not put up all the detailed headings that you do in an undergraduate lecture. You may skip the middle steps of the argument if the audience is genuinely aware of the techniques. You will certainly spend more time on the vital parts of the apparatus and on the anomalies. But it should still have the flavour of excitement. Why was the experiment designed this way? How were the measurements made? Where did that equation come from? Why did I use this catalyst? Unless the controlled excitement is present, boredom will as usual creep in. Even the listener whose work is in the same narrow field will soon find his attention wandering. Why then do the 99.9 per cent lecture as they do? Simply because they are reproducing verbatim their next publication to be. Scientific publications are not noted for their fluency.

Let's spend a bit longer watching one of these colloquia-givers in operation. Notice the abundance, the super-abundance of his slides. There's a sort of craving for showing you all his earlier work and a firm belief that you are interested. Just like holiday slides really. There will be many slides of the 'I meant to leave this one out', which he didn't, 'but as it's in, I may as well point out one or two small features' type. And small and many are the features that get pointed out. Then comes queries like 'Can we go back to the slide showing Beckenhausen's first results?' which can be hell upon earth for the projectionist who cares nothing for Beckenhausen, still less for what Beckenhausen found. And when eventually, after very many false alarms, the results of the aforementioned Beckenhausen again grace the screen, our attention is directed to a solitary point far away from the main peppering. This solitary wanderer appears to have been the source of the colloquia-giver's inspiration. To him it represents the downfall of classical biology, modern physics, theoretical chemistry, or whatever. He furiously jabs the innocent screen with the pointer as he attempts to strike the offending point. What he fails to realise is that the miscreant got there because dear befuddled old Beckenhausen happened to mix up the ordinate and abscissa of one of the points when plotting the graph. Nothing more. After Beckenhausen comes the apologetic 'I haven't had time to get a slide made of this as we only got the results this morning', which is possibly the truth. From some scrap of paper a graph is drawn which looks for all the world like everything that has gone before, or is ever likely to appear in the future. And we are meant to 'ooh-ah' in wonder at it all. How can we when the axes haven't been labelled?

By now there is a distinct air of restlessness in the theatre. It is generated by all save the two with their bulging folders and by the gentleman at the back, now in happier spheres. The would-be-up-and-coming young lecturer has been seen to look at his watch. Even the professor has ceased making gestures.

After some seventy-five minutes of his sixty the winding-up process begins. This is the most agonising part of the whole proceedings. We hear about what he hasn't got time to cover; of the experiments which his research students are working on; of the follies of his youth and of his hopes for the future. We are now told quite casually that there may have been a spanner in the works all along; so everything he has said these last ninety minutes is probably invalid. At long last, and without warning, he returns to the front row and sits down. The two with their cloth-covered folders bulging a little more offer a few claps. The professor stirs himself and, standing once more at the end of the lecture bench, confesses to being a wiser man now. (A lie! He could no more understand it than the rest of us.) He discloses that Dr Jones has said he will be happy to answer any questions.

Are there any questions? Can they be kept as brief as possible as Dr Jones must catch a train. (It's not Dr Jones who
wants to catch the train.) Dr Jones returns to the bench and
the professor hesitatingly sits down. There is silence. We
keep our fingers crossed. Then it happens. The would-be-up-
and-coming young lecturer who was seen to scribble rapidly
at one point explodes:

'Just a quick point. I wonder if perhaps I might take you
up on something you said about Beckenhausen's work and
ask whether, in comparing your results with his, you might
not just have forgotten to take into account the influence
of . . .?' It goes on and on. Battle is being engaged. He is out
to out-symposia the lecturer. He must drive home his
charge:

'Wouldn't your results have been more meaningful if
you had taken heat losses into account?'

If he knew his onions, the lecturer would realise that, for
maximum effect, the length of an answer should be in-
versely proportional to that of the question. But instead of
admitting with a 'Yes', or denying it with a 'No', he wades
in and fumbles his way through many a rubbed-out chalk
mark and many a jumbled slide as he tries to recollect just
what Beckenhausen has said or done. He is lost. The professor comes to his rescue, suggesting that the conversation
could, perhaps, be more profitably continued in private
afterwards. He again expresses very many thanks on behalf
of all and initiates a forced burst of applause, ably assisted by
the would-be-up-and-coming young lecturer.

There must be a moral here somewhere.

CHAPTER

11

Conferences

Unlike the other potential delegates the principal attraction for us of The 84th International Conference on High Temperature Physics to be held at St Andrews in August is the golf. This conference offers the only foreseeable opportunity of a golfing holiday at the tax-payer's expense, and unless the tax-payer finances it, there will be no holiday for us this year. At the same time we have every sympathy with the other delegates. How repugnant they will find the golfing climate, how alien to the physics of high temperatures. We can hear their wrath on being told the venue. We can watch their pens furiously demanding an explanation as to why Stoke or Hull was not chosen. One can only assume that the organisers did indeed try Hull and Stoke first, but that all accommodation had been reserved for delegates attending some conference on fishing or pottery. But why then have the fishermen found it necessary to congregate in the South of France this summer, and why is a ski-ing resort the only town which will extend its hospitality to the potters this winter?

Honesty being one of the hallmarks of the academic, we plan to inform the professor that we intend taking a fortnight's golfing holiday in Scotland this August at the laboratory's expense. But human weakness being an even greater hallmark of ours, we decide against the direct approach. Tact is what's required.

If there is a one hundred per cent sure way of attending a conference with the laboratory's compliments it is to read a paper. The professor has a little weakness for papers bearing his department's name and address. The weakness must be exploited. And exploit it we will. We hark back over our research; a career which is more than adequately summarised in a blue-bound thesis with its gilt lettering proclaiming 'The Fermi-Surface of the α-form of β-brass. A. J. Walton.' (Strictly speaking, the gilt lettering wasn't insisted upon by the university authorities, but I had it put on the spine to assist identification. It only cost me an extra thirty-six shillings for the four copies.) We reach up and remove the tome from its awkwardly prominent position on our shelves and open it at the Table of Contents. High temperatures, we note with much regret, are not exactly in evidence: the thesis is distressingly preoccupied with low temperatures. To further complicate matters we have already sifted three papers from these pearls. As the last of these was of necessity published in a, let's face it, obscure Chinese journal we start to doubt even our own ability to extract yet another paper. And one on high temperatures into the bargain. The tee, the number four iron, and the rough mist over before our eyes. We pull ourselves together; the search will not be abandoned as readily as this. With new grit we redirect our attention to the Contents. There must still be some cream to the milk. Chapter 3 on 'Experimental Techniques' looks the most hopeful. We turn it up and pry into its secrets. We read how we employed a furnace to prepare our specimens. We had forgotten all about this. Our spirits rise and the driver and the fairway return to view, as does the green and the putt in one. That furnace, we remember now, was inherited from someone who had done something to γ-brass; we know not what. He has since forsaken the academic world for the cloisters – he claims it's the only place where true scholarship is still to be found. We had to devote three weeks to finding out how the wretched furnace was wired up. And it took us another five to get it working properly.

With Section 3.4 before us we write our paper on 'An improved furnace for the preparation of crystals of β-brass'. Armed with the letter of acceptance from the conference referees we seek an audience with our professor. It is granted. The *fait* is *accompli*.

Despite our misgivings we do attend the opening session. We attend it for there is much to be enjoyed in the opening sessions of all conferences. Take the chairman, for example. He is a local nobody. Or rather, he is a local somebody. Very likely he is the regional professor of physics. However, his name is unknown to us. To him has been entrusted the task of welcoming us to St Andrews, Paris, Rome, or to wherever our fancy has taken us. Warm welcomes are extended from everyone who will be glad to see the back of us, and we are reminded of the last occasion the conference met here. It was in the spring of 1891. Then the local papers reported the same weather conditions as we are experiencing now. In 1891 the total number of participants was a mere two dozen, drawn from three countries. Today the assembly numbers two thousand, drawn from thirty-three nations, of which six have only recently emerged. Being unsure which heart-string these statistics are supposed to tug at, we surmise whether the level of scholarship has increased in the same sort of ratio over the years. We look about and reach our conclusions in time to hear the chairman inform us of the state of the subject way back in 1891. Although he was not around in person, he understands the electron had still to be discovered; a fact which may not have escaped the assembled masses. Then high temperature meant boiling lead. Today it means something different. We are told precisely what. We have learnt of the existence of the hydrogen bomb and of the urgency of nuclear disarmament.

After re-echoing his welcomes to all and sundry, the chairman's next honoured task is to call upon the distinguished speaker. He will be the President of the Association, the recipient of someone's medal, or an invited Duke. Riveting his attention just above the chairman's head, the distinguished speaker hears yet again that old chestnut about himself, the old chestnut which long ago was started on its travels by some journalist. The chestnut which has travelled far and wide but not very well. He manages to force yet another smile and to shake his head immodestly. He is a good seventy and all his work was carried out in the 1930s, elegant work for its time, work which has found its way into first-year undergraduate texts. We have all heard of it and are curious to see what its author looks like. He doesn't resemble his photographs, but they were probably taken years ago. For a man of his age he is still remarkably coherent. He is magnanimous in his comments, probably too much so. If I were him I wouldn't throw away suggestions for experiments so freely. Mind you, he is probably only throwing ideas around because he has quitted the labs for good. But maybe he tried them out and found they didn't work, and never published the fact. Why didn't he publish the negative results like the rest of us? Is he deliberately trying to lead us up the garden path? Come to think of it though, he would never pass our M.Sc. exams. He can be dismissed. He is dismissed as we make for the golf course.

Swiping away at our total of 127 over sixteen holes we have the nasty suspicion that we have seen our fellow golfers elsewhere. We are not entirely certain but . . . We reject the suggestion and resume our attempts at persuading the stubborn tenant of some rabbit hole to play the game, but our pleas to return the ball go unheeded. Our thoughts return to the halls of learning and to what might be happening there.

Back in the halls of learning the opening session has concluded and now it's all cheap biscuits and cups of instant coffee at five pence a time. Eager research students are running about squinting out the likes of Pippard from the name-tags. One has just published, with two others, his first of many trivial papers on something. He is on the scent of the biggest name in this something, expecting to receive a blessing, but the big name isn't up-todate. The young professors from the newer universities are busy exchanging notes on their respective empires, and growing in their own estimations. The elder statesmen are trying to recall when they last met and secretly wonder whether they will meet again this side of Paradise. Queues of persons wishing to exchange their invitations to the Lord Mayor's reception for invitations to the university reception have formed at the enquiry desk. They are quite open about it. Booking all-day tours of the Highlands is a more cloak and dagger affair. The far-sighted will have booked in advance by post.

There is a buzz or a tinkle, cups are rudely deposited on assorted ledges, and any of the two hundred who have resisted the call of the green hive off to their separate sections. The conference has now sub-divided. Each of these sections has its own president or chairman who is about to deliver his inaugural address for fifty guineas. The address will reappear as a review article, this time for eighty guineas, in the near future, and can be passed over. Merely let it be hoped that history will apportion praise differently. The lunch break follows. The delegates pick up their complimentary document cases in blue plastic with the municipal bus routes safely inside, and disperse.

We read our watches, stow our clubs, and return to our Hall of Residence. We check if the post has arrived and exchange one lunch ticket for one lunch. Over coffee, seated in a much-worn armchair, we survey the pale-faced enthusiasts digesting their conference handbooks. The handbook is bulky, distended by résumés of all the ten-minute contributions. Ours is one such, due for delivery five days from now at 15.50 hours in the theatre normally reserved for zoology but which for the duration has become room J.3. We try to guess how many of the enthusiasts are circling our names. Our contribution is listed about one-eighth of an inch in from the back cover: so we have our answer.

We theorise on why they will make a point of attending Section J next Friday at 3.50 p.m. Have they too built furnaces for growing crystals of β-brass? Have they, perhaps, published notes on their pets in *The Journal of Scientific Instruments* or written a letter to *Nature* on some obscure properly of β-brass? They will expect their contribution to be handsomely acknowledged by us and are going to be disappointed. It's not as if they have to be seen by anyone at these talks; the main sessions are the place for this. If they are genuinely interested in furnaces for growing crystals of β-brass the abstract will tell them enough, although before long it will be served up again as a proper paper embracing far more than any reasonable person could desires. If they are still disgruntled they will find out ten minutes reproduced verbatim in the 3,500-page *Proceedings of The 84th International Conference on High Temperature Physics*, to be put on sale before the year is out at twenty-five guineas. Their laboratory will surely purchase at least one copy; most probably two. That will effectively give us three papers to our credit, unless of course we find a flaw in the heater winding which will entail our writing a further note on the subject. That, if we are not mistaken, will make a grand total of four papers with which to impress the promotions committee.

Our next four and a half days are spent among the rough, while the evenings pass away amidst the smooth talk of receptions. Receptions can, however, be the happy hunting grounds for new ideas. New ideas can be plundered with great ease at receptions. You simply make out that your field is far removed from that of the innocent under interrogation. You have heard his name being proclaimed from the roof tops and are anxious to hear how he did it, although, as you have already remarked, it is not your field.

It is not enough simply to pirate the man's ideas. You must find out how far his experiments have progressed. You will not give chase unless you can beat him to it. 'Well then, where are you going to direct your attentions next? Have you thought about how you will tackle this new problem? What make of amplifier do you plan to use? How will you grow your specimens?' All is disclosed, and you may

move on to congratulate your next victim on his latest publication. Wherever would we be without conferences?

The reception-free evenings are wined and dined away
with old friends we made while attending the 82nd Conference in Delhi and the 83rd in Ontario. As we down our
coq au vin we forget how we once scolded the wife for buying
sardines in oil when pilchards in tomato are cheaper. We
have remembered to send her a postcard though; one of the
High Street taken, we guess, when the conference was last
here. It was the cheapest Woolworths could offer and has
gone second-class. By now our secretary should have received
a card painting a somewhat more colourful and, be it said,
truer picture of the conference. We drink toasts to the 85th
Conference to be held in Melbourne and to the 86th tentatively fixed for Moscow, and stumble out into the cool
night air.

Friday comes. Three-fifty p.m. comes. A buzzer dismisses
the previous speaker in Section J and a bored chairman
yawns your name and the title of your contribution. Half
the audience exits and a new half enters. You adjust the
lamp over the lectern, remove the clip from your typed
sheets and open wide your jaws. What you say matters not
a damn. You know why the audience is there. They know
why you are here. What you have to say and how you choose
to say it makes not one iota of difference.

Can anything useful be said in ten minutes? Certainly
not a repetition of what is in the handbook, nor a rehash of
the petty details deleted much against your wishes from the
abstract submitted six months ago. Nor yet what you plan
to do with the furnace should it ever reach the state you
pretend it to have reached already. Sufficient unto the day
is the evil thereof. In the course of ten minutes you may be
able to give an honest account of what has been accomplished so far. If your description serves as an *hors-d'oeuvre*
to whet the appetite for the more substantial fare to be published later you have, in some strange way, succeeded. Perhaps that's all you should aim at. It comes as no surprise to

learn that Dr G. Kitson Clark finds it necessary to number these ten-minute contributions as among those problems 'which have found me at a loss, and upon which my brother cannot help'. Commander Clark, let it be noted, 'has had considerable experience in training civil defence workers'. Training civil defence workers must have been chicken-feed.

After nine more days of golf, we return home bewildered. Why did the organisers not make wining and dining the order of the day; as well as of the night? Had they done so, the cause of true scholarship would have been advanced still further.

Ah well, back to sardines in oil.

CHAPTER

12

Facing the music

Unlike all other groups of teachers, we in higher education will receive no professional assessment of our teaching abilities, which is just as well since these professionals kept their lights firmly under bushels while we were lifting our toes off the ground. They needn't imagine they can shine them in our faces now. Ours is the harvest and we shall reap it. We will look elsewhere for advice. Our nearest and dearest; they will help. If their judgement can be relied upon we shall invite them along to criticise our lectures. If they are not completely trustworthy we will hold them at arm's length for the present. Let's begin nearer home with some thoughts on examinations. You can always tell a man by the way he conducts an examination.

Students who love quoting at you what members of The Athenaeum list as the objectives of education become quite docile over examinations. Unlike Gaul or detergent packagings, all students see examinations as divided simply into the 'wasn't too bad' and the 'b—y awful' categories. Set a paper in the first category and you can very profitably waltz around the campus smiling benignly at all and sundry. Set one in the second category and you will pursue the shortest route from A to B. Of course you have quite deliberately set a 'b—y awful' paper because the class played up and you are determined to demonstrate just who is the winner; square up to them if you have. There is no real knack to setting such a paper – it comes quite naturally after a term's lecturing. Because you haven't had time to cover the required material you will whitewash this failure by asking questions on the missing topics. This creates the right illusion with those who matter.

Students, returning spic and span from their mother's attentions, take their place in the Examination Hall. Like a general inspecting his troops you parade up and down the rows plonking down one or more paper on each desk. Behind you their disbelieving eyes scan and rescan the pages – they are all brothers in adversity. Some half-dozen protest that you have given them the wrong paper and you half convince them that you haven't. You announce that the paper is a three hour one and they all swap looks. Eventually there is peace and they settle down to draw match stick men in the margins, or to writing verbose essays on such irrelevancies as 'Inorganic Compounds' while you, up front, feel well satisfied with all the ink-work in progress. Comes marking time and the note of pleasure is only held by scaling all the marks up by a factor of 3.5. Now is the hour to congratulate yourself on the results. You may have fooled your professor, but you can't fool students that easily.

To impress students you must set a 'not too bad' paper; one in which the average chap confidently expects sixty per cent, and on which an egg-head knows he won't be mistaken as a pin-head, because of an inadequate spread in marks. Almost any muggins can set a paper which produces a high average mark; you repeat effectively the same paper year in and year out; you limit the questions to well-defined topics more satisfactorily discussed in the textbooks than you managed in lectures, or you set such nebulous essays (' "The cell is the nucleus". Discuss') that students couldn't possibly anticipate their marks. To introduce the element of discrimination is more difficult. Now for the sixty-four-thousand-dollar question: who, or what, should we dis-discriminate between? Between the healthy and the ill; between the fast and the slow writer, between the critical and credulous; between those who can remember definitions and those who don't bother; between those who can extrapolate and those who can't even interpolate. You should have made up your own mind months ago on which of these opposing attitudes to wear. The attitudes you donned this past term will, in part, be theirs now; there is therefore no point in probing for many fresh qualities in an examination. How best to search out a student's qualities will require another volume. Any trite answer such as suggesting you adopt 'objective multichoice questions' may do the cause more harm than good. Instead of setting that general essay on 'Myriapods' you may now ask the class 'Has a centipede (a) 10 legs, (b) 100 legs, (c) 1,000 legs or (d) none of these?' Such multichoice questions may, all too easily, simply reflect your own unhealthy state and give the student little opportunity to exhibit superior attitudes. Many a don setting an 'objective' examination puts his feet up once he finds that the class's marks lie on a good-looking histogram. He will announce that he has reached the seventh heaven, forgetting that he could have obtained the same result by playing darts in a pub. Until you know where you are heading, stick to the well-tried cocktails. But let's return to examining our own particular strengths.

We are, after all, self-made men free to indulge in a little self-criticism. We will. We will compare the new man with the old. Just contrast the confident air with which we now fling wide those theatre doors with the shame-faced struggles of three months ago. Observe the almost clinical skill we have acquired in dislodging a paper-clip; yesterday it was a reluctant wrestle. Today we remove a piece of chalk from the box in one fell swoop, a full-length stick which is proudly held aloft. We have arrived.

Not so fast. As soon as a lecture is over, read your notes through exactly as you intended them to be delivered. Compare your intentions with what went on the board. Hang around waiting to be asked embarrassing questions. Sneak a look at a set of notes taken in your lecture. It will be clear what went wrong. Very much went wrong. Now make a little list of your failings. Take your little list into the next lecture and leave it on the bench. There you will read such telling reminders as 'Look at the class. Ask them questions. Write up only what's planned. Omit nothing planned. Don't side-track'. As the pop psychologists warn, before many weeks have passed your list will shrink. Which proves just about anything.

How about taping one of your lectures? Do, and you will be able to spot your overworked phrases, your bat-like voice and your wrong emphases. You will discover that you also 'er' and 'um'. Or you may decide that the speed and style of your delivery are better suited to a political meeting than to an university lecture. All you lack is the politician's facility to sound sincere, and maybe to win converts. And what about those juicy asides in the audience? Surely they can't all have been meant for your ears? Now try taping a tutorial. You will soon learn who talks too much.

Of course, you are laughing if you are fortunate enough to be able to have your lectures video-recorded. Now, one would think that, in view of the agony experienced with the sound-analysis, when vision is added it would be more than any ordinary mortal could bear. But not a bit of it. There is a strange something in everyone which emerges when they watch themselves on telly. Lecturers who by any standard touch rock-bottom have been heard to remark, on watching the playback, that they now know as a truth that no one on Broadway touches them in style, delivery, or in any other grace revealed to man. It wears off though. Second time round some small doubts will be raised about the finer points of style. Third time round less finer points will be questioned. Fourth time round they will spot they have filthy personal habits. Let them keep it up. Unless they do they will be left puzzling over why they are not earning £2,000 a week at the B.B.C. instead of £30 in their present job.

As we grow in self-confidence we can, with impunity, remove our nearest and dearest from cold storage and tell them frantically, desperately, that we need their help. The sort of help they alone can give, the help we will treasure till our dust to dust. Just what would they do if they were in our shoes? And you, knowing your nearest and dearest as you do, will know exactly how to interpret it.

If there is one group who are for ever ready to offer criticism of us, or anyone else in range, it is our own dear students. Strong meaty criticism; the venom that flows gratuitously through the columns of student newspapers. Ah well, critique writers aren't typical. Of course, if we choose to ask the right student we will be absolved from all responsibility. Our inability to operate a projector can be traced to our membership of the bourgeoisie or to our wrong party ticket. Only when all is finally overthrown will be be able to thread up that 16mm machine. Roll on The Revolution.

Some student criticism is very pointed; they get up and walk out. Should this happen to one of us we will know that all is not well. Now it may simply be that we have walked into a room-full expecting an hour on 'The Role of Shakespeare in Anglo-Sino Relations' and we have offered them 'Second-Order Partial Differential Equations'. My own advice is that, should this ever happen to you, get up and walk out also. Stay put and you will be tempted to show how second-order partial differential equations may be applied to Shakespeare. You will struggle around with some partial-differential equation for unstrained mercy, with rather unhappy results. Should you continue to make this particular sort of mistake, then do seek the help which no student need ever fear to seek.

We have seen the perils of being insensitive to criticism. Better scoop up all we can ere it's too late. We will stand up and ask to be told all. We are men, and we can take it. Tell us and we will mend our ways. Better not, actually. Well, perhaps we could suggest that if there are any little criticisms they might care to send us anonymous notes. Only cranks write. So, and this is where the twentieth-century methods break in with all their glory, we will give each a fifty-page questionnaire and beg him to spend ten hours answering questions about us. The answers will be fed into computers by statisticians. The results will be analysed by sociologists, economists and anthropologists. Six months later they will notify us that our material has been poorly thought out, we have not been observing the class, that our use of the blackboard has been erratic, our vocal techniques need improving, and that fifty per cent of the class say we go too slowly and fifty per cent too fast. And it won't make any difference if the questionnaire is five hundred pages long or if the university does get that new computer which is needed to handle the increasing volume of work – the conclusions will be the same.

Which is more or less where you and I came in.

BIBLIOGRAPHY

BEARD, R. *Teaching and Learning in Higher Education*. London: Penguin Books, 1970. A rigorous analysis of existing university teaching techniques. Not for beginners!

BIDDER CLARK, E. and KITSON CLARK, G. *The Art of Lecturing*. Cambridge: Heffer, 1959. Practical hints directed at the arts man.

BLOOM, B. S. (Ed.) *Taxonomy of Educational Objectives 1: Cognitive Domain*. New York: Longmans, Green, 1956. The standard work on the subject. Gives all the jargon.

LAYTON, D. (Ed.) *University Teaching in Transition*. Edinburgh: Oliver and Boyd, 1968. A collection of papers reviewing the effectiveness of present methods of teaching.

ROGERS, J. (Ed.) *Teaching on Equal Terms*. London: British Broadcasting Corporation, 1969. Primarily concerned with extra-mural adult education. Practical.

UNIVERSITY GRANTS COMMITTEE. *Report of the Committee on University Teaching Methods*. London: H.M.S.O., 1964. Spells out the functions of lectures, seminars, colloquia, etc.

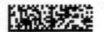